Study Guide

for the

Therapeutic Recreation Specialist Certification Examination

Third Edition

Norma J. Stumbo
Jean E. Folkerth

Sagamore Publishing, L.L.C.

Production coordinator: Janet Wahlfeldt
Interior design: Jeff Higgerson
Cover design: Jeff Higgerson

ISBN: 1-57167-554-x
Library of Congress Catalog Card Number: 2004097927

http://www.sagamorepub.com

10 9 8

Contents

ACKNOWLEDGMENTS   V

SECTION ONE

CHAPTER ONE
Introduction to the Study Guide 1
 Purpose of the Study Guide 2
 How to Use the Study Guide 2

CHAPTER TWO
What Is Competence and How Is It Measured? 4
 Validity, Reliability and Fairness 5
 How Was the NCTRC Exam Developed? 6
 How Has the Revised NCTRC Test Changed? 6
 References 7

CHAPTER THREE
Strategies for Preparing and Taking the Test 8
 Preparing for the Test 8
 Taking the Test 10
 References 11

CHAPTER FOUR
Basic Information on the Test Content Outline 12
 Introduction 12
 Background 15
 Diagnostic Groupings and Populations Served 23
 Assessment 31
 Planning the Intervention 35
 Implementing the Individualized Intervention Plan 43
 Documentation and Evaluation 48
 Organizing and Managing Services 52
 Advancement of the Profession 57

SECTION TWO

CHAPTER FIVE
Warm-Up Items 70

CHAPTER SIX
Practice Tests 92

CHAPTER SEVEN
Diagnostic and Review Items 134

About the Authors. . .

NORMA J. STUMBO received her B.S. and M.S. in Recreation and Park Administration/ Therapeutic Recreation from the University of Missouri-Columbia and her Ph.D. in Leisure Studies/Therapeutic Recreation from the University of Illinois at Urbana-Champaign. She is currently a professor of therapeutic recreation at Illinois State University in Normal, Illinois. Dr. Stumbo served on the Board of Directors of the National Council for Therapeutic Recreation Certification from 1981 to 1989, serving as Chair of the Test Management Committee from 1982 to 1989 and Vice President from 1988 to 1989. She has authored over 200 publications and conducted over 400 presentations at the local, state, and national levels, on a variety of topics, including entry-level knowledge, curriculum, assessment, evaluation, and leisure education.

JEAN E. FOLKERTH received her B.S. in Camping and Outdoor Education/Therapeutic Recreation from Indiana University, her M.A. in Therapeutic Recreation from Michigan State University, and her Re.D. in Recreation Administration/Therapeutic Recreation from Indiana University. She is currently an associate professor and director of the Recreation Therapy Program at the University of Findlay in Findlay, Ohio. Dr. Folkerth served on the Board of Directors of the National Council for Therapeutic Recreation Certification from 1984 to 1989, serving as president from 1985 to 1987. She served on the Board of Directors of the National Therapeutic Recreation Society from 1979 to 1982 and was instrumental in the implementation of the State and Regional Advisory Council for NTRS. Currently, Dr. Folkerth is co-chair of the Alliance Taskforce on Higher Education representing the American Therapeutic Recreation Association. Dr. Folkerth has authored several publications and conducted over 100 presentations at state, regional, and national levels on topics including credentialing, professional preparation, and professional issues.

Acknowledgments

We would like to acknowledge several individuals who have helped with this publication. First, we would like to thank Dr. Marcia J. Carter from the University of Northern Colorado. We benefit greatly from her expertise.

We also owe thanks to the many individuals who used the second edition and let us know what they thought about it. Their comments have helped to improve the third edition. We hope the audience of the third edition feels equally free to share their advice about the *Study Guide*.

Our students have also helped us clarify ideas and questions, with ideas and questions of their own. We appreciate their comments on draft versions, as well as on individual items. In addition, their patience with our absences from campus to hide away and write are appreciated. May you all achieve above the cut scores!

We also appreciate the support of our families and partners.

The staff at Sagamore Publishing has been exceptional. We appreciate the support and enthusiasm of their efforts.

SECTION ONE

Chapter One
Introduction to the Study Guide

Welcome to the third edition of the *Study Guide for the Therapeutic Recreation Specialist Certification Examination*! We are excited to tell you that the third edition (2005) has changed significantly from the second edition (1997) and the first edition (1990).

The third edition has 90 warm-up items—40 more than the second edition, and *two* practice tests—instead of just one. Like the second edition, there are 240 diagnostic and review items that focus on specific areas, if you have trouble with the two practice tests.

As always, the absolute best information about the NCTRC exam comes from the *NCTRC Candidate Bulletin*. More detailed information about the exam—which is now computerized—such as when and where it is administered, and sitting requirements in order to qualify to take the exam are available at:

National Council for Therapeutic
    Recreation Certification
7 Elmwood Drive
New City, NY 10956
Telephone: 845 639-1439
Fax: 845 639-1471
Website: www.NCTRC.org

Section One of this *Study Guide* includes the following four chapters:

- Chapter One:
  Introduction to the Study Guide.

- Chapter Two:
  What is Competence and How is It Measured?

- Chapter Three:
  Strategies for Preparing and Taking the Test.

- Chapter Four:
  Basic Information about the Test Content.

Section Two of this *Study Guide*:

- Chapter Five:
  Warm Up Items (90 items)

- Chapter Six:
  Practice Test 1 (90 items)
  Practice Test 2 (90 items)

- Chapter Seven:
  Diagnostic and Review Items (240 items)

Purpose of the Study Guide

The purpose of this *Study Guide* is to assist candidates in preparing for the National Council for Therapeutic Recreation Certification's (NCTRC) national certification examination for Therapeutic Recreation Specialists. The *Study Guide's* mission is two-fold: a.) to provide information on reducing test anxiety and improving test performance; and b.) to provide numerous sample questions, similar to those actually found on the exam, which will allow candidates to practice and self-assess their own readiness for the test.

We have tried to provide enough background information to give you some idea of what to expect when you take or "sit" for the exam. Every attempt has been made to make this *Study Guide* both usable and "user friendly." We hope you will find it both a valuable resource and a learning tool. This *Study Guide* is meant to be used in conjunction with the *NCTRC Candidate Bulletin,* which provides very specific information about registering for and taking the national exam.

For many individuals, the thought of taking a certification examination can be unsettling. We often hear statements like, "I have never taken a comprehensive exam, there is so much information. How do I learn it all?" or "I've been out of school for ten years, how do I go about studying for the test?" Be assured that many of your colleagues across the nation have the same types of questions that you do. These kinds of questions, and others, hopefully will be answered by reading and completing this *Study Guide*.

We have tried to provide you with a condensed but complete set of materials. We trust that you will find the information and resources contained in the *Study Guide* to be helpful in getting ready for the national examination.

How to Use the Study Guide

We advise that you read the first four chapters before going to the sample test questions. The first three provide background information. You may find the third chapter helpful at several points in your own preparation.

The fourth chapter is important in that it gives you information about what will be on the test. The NCTRC Content Outline represents the result of several NCTRC committees working in conjunction with Educational Testing Service (ETS) and lays the foundation for the examination. The Content Outline contains eight areas, that are represented on the test. In our overview, we give you an idea of what information comes from each of the eight areas, as well as references to scrutinize if some content sounds unfamiliar to you. **Study the Content Outline and accompanying information thoroughly.** This is the most complete information you will receive about what will be on the test.

Before we go further, we want to clarify an important point. The format used for the items is nearly identical to that used by NCTRC and ETS to develop the national certification test. However, do not expect to see the same items on the actual NCTRC test. **The items in these chapters represent similar format and content as the NCTRC exam, but this does not mean they are the same items found on the test.** Keep in mind that these are practice items.

The sample test items are divided into three chapters. The first is a set of 90 "warm-up" items that you may want to use if it has been a while since you have taken a multiple-choice test. Familiarize yourself with the style of the items and get back into the feel of taking a test. The content was randomly selected from all eight areas of the Content Outline. A scoring sheet is provided at the end of this chapter.

The second chapter in this section provides two complete practice tests that mimic the proportions of the actual test. We have developed items in the same proportional amounts as you will find on the actual exam. (For example, out of the 90 items, the area of Assessment has about 14 items.) More information about the percentages of items on the actual test is found in Chapter Four: Background Information.

We suggest you sit and take Practice Test 1 in one sitting, to get the feel of how you will fare physically and mentally during the actual test. While we cannot copy the real testing environment, especially since computers are used, we want you to get a notion of how physical and mental fatigue may affect you. If this is significant, you may want to review the chapter on Strategies for Test Preparation.

A scoring key is provided at the end of Practice Test 1, and should help you determine if you need to move on to Practice Test 2. A second answer sheet and scoring key are provided for Practice Test 2.

The scoring keys provide more detailed diagnostic information about which parts of the Content Outline you did well on, and which you did not. If there is one or more areas in which you did not do well, you may want to move on to the third chapter of items.

Depending on your scores for either or both exams, you may want to progress on to the third chapter in this section. The Diagnostic and Review Items cover each of the eight areas, with 30 questions each.

The purpose of the third chapter in this section is to give you even more practice taking items concerning certain content areas. Each of the eight areas is clearly labeled, with 30 items per area. Again, we remind you that these identical items will not be found on the actual NCTRC test. But if you find that you miss several items, say concerning documentation and goal writing, you will know this is an area on which you should concentrate your efforts before you sit for the national exam.

Remember, the *Study Guide* is meant to be a framework to help you prepare for and to let you know what to expect on the test. You may use it as a diagnostic tool of sorts to learn the areas where you need more preparation.

Chapter Two
What Is Competence and How Is It Measured?

Competence is a goal of all professionals. It is achieved not only through structured professional preparation programs or through workshops and conferences. It is not automatically granted on graduation day or at the one-year anniversary date on our first job. Competence is a never-ending, far-reaching concept that affects our practice, our livelihood, and our profession. To master one's responsibilities in a competent fashion takes considerable effort, learning and patience. It is not to be taken lightly as consumers. The public and our colleagues depend on us to be competent in practice. Competence is a full-time job.

As such, competence is sometimes difficult to define and most literature identifies three concerns with its definition. The first concern is that it is often too complex and difficult, with all of our job responsibilities, to say whether one is competent or not, when the job is viewed as a whole. Often, it is easier to view it as a set of "competencies"—that is, individual, but interrelated tasks that are performed on the job (Olson & Freeman, 1979). This definition becomes more workable because we can derive a list of specific and important areas or competencies of professional practice. This delineation of separate components allows for the measurement of each area as well as the whole. We depend upon separate components of the job to define and measure the entire job. "These components must be identified as they relate to the individual's ability to achieve positive professional practice outcomes, particularly positive client outcomes" (Scofield, Berven & Harrison, 1981, p. 34). We will discuss more specifics about the competencies expected in therapeutic recreation when we discuss the NCTRC Content Outline in chapter four.

The second concern in measuring competence is whether we look at the applicant's *potential* for competence or the *performance* of some specified tasks (Olson & Freeman, 1979). The major question here is whether competence may be verified before or after the behavior is demonstrated. In a testing situation, the difference is whether you have the knowledge of how a hypothetical procedure would be applied versus demonstrating that you can perform the actual procedure (Stumbo, 1989). For example, in first-aid procedures, there is a difference in whether you are asked to list on paper the steps of cardiopulmonary resuscitation versus actually performing the procedures on an inflatable dummy. The first method looks at your *potential* to apply the procedures, the second asks you to *perform* the procedures. The potential/performance debate becomes more important as the profession has an increased potential or capacity to harm clients. For example, we would all want surgeons to actually demonstrate their surgical abilities rather than just their knowledge of surgical procedures. However, for most professions, testing the individual's demonstration of a skill is impractical, because it is too time consuming and expensive. Most professions choose to test the individual's potential through paper and pencil or computerized examinations.

The third, closely related concern in measuring competence is whether the test measures the applicant's knowledge or skills of application. The major question here is the level required by the job. For each of the important competencies, the question asked is whether the competent professional needs a basic knowledge or thorough understanding with the ability to apply this to a given situation (Shimberg, 1981). For example, in therapeutic recreation, is it more appropriate to be able to list available assessment instruments or to be able to apply the process of collecting client information for programming purposes? The latter seems more appropriate to ensure competence practice. Most questions on the exam will ask the candidate to apply the information to a practice situation.

All three of these issues focus on the idea of job-relatedness. Above all else, the examination developers must demonstrate that the basic structure and items of the exam are valid, reliable and fair. These characteristics combine to create the degree of job-relatedness of the examination—how closely do the knowledges and skills of the test match those required by the job? This concept is extremely important in certification examinations. If the

basic purpose is to attest to the certificant's competence, then the test has to be an accurate, dependable, and equitable measure of professional competence.

Validity, Reliability and Fairness

Let's look further at the concepts of validity, reliability, and fairness. A brief explanation of these concepts will help you understand the process used in conducting the national job analysis and certification test specifications.

Validity determines whether the test measures what it is intended to measure (Gronlund, 1981). If the test is intended to measure competence in professional therapeutic recreation practice, does it do that? How well does it measure the knowledge, skills, and abilities necessary for minimal competence in entry-level practice?

Most testing organizations use content validation as the overall approach for determining the validity of the certification examination (Oltman, Norback, & Rosenfeld, 1989). There are psychometric standards that outline the processes to be used, but basically, content validation involves the use of expert panels and resources (such as literature and job descriptions) to determine and refine the contents of the test. The use of these avenues helps ensure that the test is measuring what it is intended to measure—that is, minimal professional competence.

Reliability refers to the consistency or accuracy of the measurement results (Gronlund, 1981). In credentialing tests, reliability indices report how consistent results are from one administration to another as well as how accurately the results of the test relate to the job in question. If the applicant took the test twice, would he or she score approximately the same score? Is the test dependable over time? Can the test distinguish between those who are competent and those who are not?

Fairness, or non-discrimination of protected classes, is a less tangible concept but attempts to make each applicant "equal" regardless of gender, racial or ethnic background, age or similar characteristics (Educational Testing Service, 1987; Shimberg, 1987). All tests developed by the Educational Testing Service undergo "sensitivity reviews" by experts to reduce or eliminate inappropriate and potentially offensive content. In addition, every effort possible is made by the examination committees and the Educational Testing Service to eliminate test questions that appear to discriminate unfairly among different groups of test takers. The combination of professional sensitivity review and statistical analysis (differential item functioning) are very effective in guarding against potential unfairness.

How Was the NCTRC Exam Developed?

It is easy to see that there are numerous "behind-the-scenes" concerns for credentialing organizations, such as the National Council for Therapeutic Recreation Certification. Developing a national certification test that adequately defines and measures professional competence is not an easy task. The NCTRC and the Educational Testing Service have taken the task of developing and reconstructing the test quite seriously and have adhered to strict test development procedures.

How Has the Revised NCTRC Test Changed?

Note that while the same eight basic areas are found both on the original and revised Content Outlines, the percentages of weight given to each area have changed, as have some details of the content covered.

Changes in the NCTRC Test Content Outlines

1990 Test Outline

I.	Background	(8%)
II.	Diagnostic Groupings and Populations Served	(13%)
III.	Assessment	(15%)
IV.	Planning the Program/Treatment	(18%)
V.	Implementing the Program/Treatment	(16%)
VI.	Documentation and Evaluation	(9%)
VII.	Organizing and Managing Services	(10%)
VIII.	Professional Issues	(11%)

1996 Revised Outline

I.	Background	(8%)
II.	Diagnostic Groupings and Populations Served	(14%)
III.	Assessment	(14%)
IV.	Planning the Intervention	(20%)
V.	Implementing the Individual Intervention Plan	(21%)
VI.	Documentation and Evaluation	(13%)
VII.	Organizing and Managing Services	(6%)
VIII.	Advancement of the Profession	(4%)

2004 Revised Outline

I.	Background	(8%)
II.	Diagnostic Groupings and Populations Served	(15%)
III.	Assessment	(15%)
IV.	Planning the Intervention	(15%)
V.	Implementing the Individual Intervention Plan	(16%)
VI.	Documentation and Evaluation	(15%)
VII.	Organizing and Managing Services	(9%)
VIII.	Advancement of the Profession	(7%)

These changes are important to you because they change the emphasis of items on the test. Remember that chapter four provides you with more detailed information about these changes and the content covered under each area.

References

Gronlund, N.E. (1981). *Measurement and evaluation in teaching* (4th ed.). New York: MacMillan Publishing Co.

Educational Testing Service. (1986). *ETS sensitivity review process: Guidelines and procedures.* Princeton, NJ: Author.

Educational Testing Service. (1987). *ETS standards for quality and fairness.* Princeton, NJ: Author.

National Council for Therapeutic Recreation Certification. (2004). *Candidate Bulletin.* New City, NY: Author.

Olson, P.A., & Freeman, L. (1979). Defining competence in teacher licensing usage. In P. S. Pottinger, & J. Goldsmith (Eds.), *Defining and measuring competence* (pp. 1-11). San Francisco: Jossey-Bass, Inc.

Oltman, P. K., Norback, J., & Rosenfeld, M. (1989). A national study of the profession of therapeutic recreation specialist. *Therapeutic Recreation Journal,* (2), 49-58.

Scofield, M. E., Berven, N. L., & Harrison, R. P. (1981). Competence, credentialing and the future of rehabilitation. *Journal of Rehabilitation, 47*(1), 31-35.

Shimberg, B. (1981). Testing for licensure and certification. *American Psychologist, 36* (10), 1138-1146.

Shimberg, B. (1987, September/October). Assuring the continued competence of health professionals. *The Journal,* 8-14.

Stumbo, N. J. (1989). Credentialing in therapeutic recreation: Issues in ensuring the minimal competence of professionals. In D. Compton (Ed.), *Issues in therapeutic recreation: A profession in transition* (pp. 67-86). Champaign, IL: Sagamore Publishing.

Chapter Three
Strategies for Preparing and Taking the Test

This section of the *Study Guide* is divided into two major sections: Preparing for the Test and Taking the Test. Each section contains helpful hints to assist you while you are studying and sitting for the exam. The exam consists entirely of multiple-choice questions, and these strategies are based on that fact.

Overall, one major way to improve your test score is to become as familiar as possible with the test content. Read the Content Outline and chapter four (and other related materials) thoroughly. Use the sample items found in section two to practice and self-diagnose your weaker areas. The second major way to improve your test score is to improve your test taking skills. That is, becoming more "test wise." Often, a person's score may be reduced simply because he or she makes errors in recording answers, eliminating wrong answer options, and leaving questions blank. While the other sections of this *Study Guide* attempt to help you become familiar with the test content, this section deals exclusively with reviewing test-taking strategies, helping you become more "test wise."

The hint you might find most helpful in this process is to relax and enjoy it as much as possible. If nothing else, you will exit the test-ing center knowing just a bit more about the profession than when you entered, and that benefits everyone.

Preparing for the Test

1. **Start early.** If possible, give yourself at least one to two months to study before taking the exam. This time can be used for reviewing the job analysis and content outline information, looking up new or unfamiliar information, ordering necessary materials, and reviewing your notes.

2. **Review the knowledge areas within the Content Outline and complete the sample test questions.** If you have concerns about your comprehension in any area, complete the Diagnostic/Review questions in chapter seven, and review the suggested materials listed in chapter four.

3. **Do not assume that you know everything about the knowledge areas that is necessary, based on your performance on these sample questions.** We have provided the questions for your practice, but they are not exhaustive or definitive of the material covered on the exam.

This *Study Guide* is only a start; your thorough preparation is up to you.

4. **Determine how you study best.** Some individuals seem to learn better when they hear the information, while others need to see written materials, and still others prefer to discuss material with colleagues. A combination of these alternatives often can produce the most effective study patterns. We suggest you review the material individually, and then, use groups of colleagues for discussion and brainstorming of material.

5. **You might consider using note cards to jot down important or new information in categories for each of the knowledge areas.** This may help you organize your study materials. Prepare a note card or two for each knowledge area and then under each heading list relevant information as thoughtfully and concisely as possible. It also may help you to keep track of reference materials on the note cards so if questions arise later, you will be able to track down the information more quickly.

6. **Concentrate your efforts.** If you have not opened a textbook or journal for some time, this is not the time to try to catch up and read all the available material. Concentrate on a few well-chosen references from the reference list. Note which references are used repeatedly throughout chapter four. Also concentrate on the knowledge areas which have been listed as most important to practice, according to the Content Outline. These areas are the focal point for the exam content and should provide direction for your study sessions. Remember to look at the percentages of weight for each area, to know how many questions will be asked per area.

7. **Do not hesitate to call on colleagues.** Use them both as content experts and as study partners to discuss the content covered by the test. This will be helpful to all parties. Perhaps your study group might contain colleagues who work with a variety of populations in various settings. You might find it helpful to compare the practice of therapeutic recreation in diverse settings applied to different populations. Do remember to look for similarities rather than differences in practice. The job analysis revealed that there was overwhelming consensus on the sub-categories of the knowledge areas so material applicable across settings will be most useful to review. Your group may also find it helpful to create your own sample test times and review them as a group.

8. **Use whatever test anxiety you may have positively instead of negatively.** Use this energy to make the test a positive, rather than negative, experience. Think of the benefits of updating and reviewing your knowledge and focus on the larger picture of competent practice. Always ask yourself "How does this information apply to practice? How can I use this information to benefit my clients? How can I use this information in the future?"

9. **Eat sensibly and get plenty of rest the night before the test to make sure you are at your physical best.** Dress comfortably, perhaps in layers so that you can adjust to the temperature of the room if you need to.

10. **Your absolute best strategy is to be as prepared as possible for the test.** Study well in advance, feel confident with your level of knowledge, and then relax.

Taking the Test

1. **Arrive at your test site around 30 minutes early.** Do not bring friends or relatives with you as they will not be allowed to sit in the waiting room while you are taking the exam.

2. **When you arrive at the testing site the following activities will occur:**
    a. You will be asked to present photo-bearing identification that also has your signature and a second form of identification that also has your signature.
    b. You will be asked to sign in at the center and that signature will be compared to the presented identification.

    You will not be allowed to bring any items into the testing room other than your two forms of identification.

3. **You will then be escorted to a computer terminal.** The test administrator will give you a packet of scratch paper that you may use as needed. It must be given to the test administrator when you leave.

4. **A brief on-line tutorial to guide you on how to use the computer for the exam will be provided.** The tutorial will familiarize you with selecting answers, using the testing features, using the mouse, and the overall operation of the keyboard. The tutorial is a "one-time deal." Make sure you understand how to mark the answers and operate the system since once you exit the tutorial, you may not return to it.

5. **Read each test question carefully.** For each question, study the statement of the question (or item stem). Before you look at the choices, try to answer the question in your own words. Then look at the choices very carefully, not trying to find out what is right about them, but studying them to find what is wrong. Eliminate all choices that are obviously wrong or implausible, and there should always be one choice that is either obviously correct or that is the least wrong. Do make sure you read through all the answer options; do not select the first one that sounds appropriate. For example, even if option A sounds correct, be sure to read through options B, C, and D. Choose the best possible answer for that question. There will be no trick questions on the test, so try not to "read too much" into a question.

6. **Bypass those questions which you are unsure of, marking them as a reminder to review them later.** You are able to move back and forth within the base test, but the base test may not be reviewed once it has been exited. Do not go back and reconsider marked answers, trying to second guess your first-choice answers. Most likely you were right the first time and will be changing a correct answer.

7. **The NCTRC examination is what is referred to as a "variable-length" examination.** The base test consists of 90 questions for which you have 86 minutes. This is plenty of time to easily complete the test. For best results, pace yourself by periodically checking your progress. Set a pace that will allow you to make any necessary adjustments to unanswered questions. Work as quickly as you can, without being careless.

8. **Be sure to record an answer for each question, even the ones you are not completely confident of.** Make informed guesses rather than omitting items. Eliminate as many alternatives as possible on multiple-choice items before guessing. There will be no penalty for guessing.

9. **Throughout the test, remind yourself to combat any emotional responses with self-statements, such as: "Just relax; I am in control; concentrate on doing well on this exam."** Sometimes we are our own worst critic, and in a testing situation this self-criticism may have a more negative than positive effect.

10. **At the end of the base test (90 questions) you will receive**
    a. a passing score ending the exam;
    b. a failing score ending the exam; or
    c. a score that falls in the range of neither failing nor passing.

    If you received "c., a score that falls in the range of neither failing nor passing," you will move on to another section. These additional sections are called "testlets." These "testlets" will focus on the specific knowledge area for which the computer was unable to determine if you really know or don't know the material. These "testlets" each contain 15 questions and you have up to 14 minutes to complete the testlet. You may be given more than one testlet. Keep in mind that, like the "base test," once you exit the testlet, you cannot go back.

    At the end of the testlet you will once again receive
    a. a passing score ending the exam;
    b. a failing score ending the exam; or
    c. a score that falls in the range of neither passing nor failing.

If you receive the base test and all the testlets, you will complete 180 test items and a total of 180 minutes of "seat time."

You can do very well without answering every multiple-choice question or answering every time correctly. You are not expected to get a perfect score. Remember, this test covers the minimal entry-level knowledge needed for competent practice.

References

Anatasi, A. (1954). *Psychological testing.* New York: MacMillan Publishing Company.

Bergmen, J. (1981). *Understanding educational measurement and evaluation.* Boston, MA: Houghton Mifflin Company.

Drummond, R. J. (1988). *Appraisal procedures for counselors and helping professionals.* Columbus, OH: Merrill Publishing Company.

Kaplan, R. M., & Saccuzzo, D. P. (1982). *Psychological testing: Principles, applications and issues.* Monterey, CA: Brooks Cole Publishing.

National Council for Therapeutic Recreation Certification. (2004). *Candidate bulletin.* Available: [on-line] at www.nctrc.org

Chapter Four
Basic Information on the Test Content Outline

The purpose of this chapter is to provide more detailed information about the content that will be on the national certification test. This section will act as a guide through the eight different NCTRC Knowledge Areas. Its intent is to clarify concepts and to provide resources that may help you study more effectively and be better prepared for the national exam. At the end of each section is a list of resources that can be used to review more thoroughly a specific concept, if you feel you need more information.

Introduction

The original NCTRC job analysis project results in 1989-1990 presented information about nine major job responsibilities and eight major knowledge areas. While the second job analysis was conducted for the new edition of the NCTRC test, the original job responsibilities and knowledge areas did not change significantly for the current test. The primary changes in the knowledge areas were in the titles and the percentage weights of specific knowledge areas in the overall test. There was minimal change in the overall content, although some shifting of areas occurred. In the third revision, again, only minimal changes in the knowledge areas were made. Thus, one can assume that the information necessary to be an entry-level therapeutic recreation specialist has remained relatively stable in the last 15 year.

The job analysis essentially was the blueprint for the development of the national exam. Before the development of the test took place, the content outline was developed based on the knowledge areas, with weights (approximate number of test items included on each topic) identified for each knowledge area. The test was developed based on this content outline. Table 1 presents the NCTRC Knowledge Areas accompanied by their prevalence on the test.

Table 2 presents the NCTRC Content Outline that is used as a guide for the remainder of this chapter. It also establishes a basis for reviewing the material covered within each category as well as providing general references for concepts and material. At the end of this chapter is a complete reference list with ISBN numbers included, so materials can be ordered directly from the publisher if they cannot be located at your local or university library or bookstore.

Table 1
NCTRC Knowledge Areas

I. Background	8%
II. Diagnostic Groupings and Populations Served	15%
III. Assessment	15%
IV. Planning the Intervention	15%
V. Implementing the Individual Intervention Plan	16%
VI. Documentation and Evaluation	15%
VII. Organizing and Managing Services	9%
VIII. Advancement of the Profession	7%

(NCTRC, 1997, p. 5)

Table 2
NCTRC Exam Content Outline*

Background   **(8 %)**

1. Human growth and development throughout the lifespan
2. Theories of human behavior change
3. Diversity factors (e.g., social, cultural, educational, language, spiritual, financial, age, attitude, geographics)
4. Recreation, leisure and play:
    a. Theories and concepts
    b. Models of service delivery
    c. Social psychological aspects
    d. Leisure throughout the lifespan
    e. Leisure lifestyle development
5. Therapeutic recreation:
    a. Concepts (e.g., holistic approach, recreative experience)
    b. Models of service delivery (e.g., special recreation, leisure ability/TR service model, activity therapy, Health & Wellness model)
    c. Historical development
    d. Practice settings
6. Service delivery systems:
    a. Health care
    b. Leisure services
    c. Education and human services systems
7. Models of health care and human services (e.g., medical model, community model, education model, psychosocial rehabilitation model, health and wellness model, person-centered model)

Diagnostic Groupings and Populations Served (Etiology, symptomatology, diagnosis, prognosis and treatment of conditions, disabilities, and related secondary complications).

(15 %)

8. Cognitive Impairments (e.g., dementia, traumatic brain injury, developmental/learning disabilities)
9. Physical Impairments (e.g., impairments in musculoskeletal system, nervous system, circulatory system, respiratory system; endocrine and metabolic disorders; infectious diseases)
10. Sensory and Communication Impairments (visual, hearing and speech)
11. Psychiatric Impairments (e.g., psychoses, affective disorders, personality disorders, polysubstance dependence, alcohol dependence, eating disorders)
12. Behavioral Impairments (e.g., victims and/or perpetrators of violence, abuses or neglect)
13. Addictions (e.g., substance abuse, eating disorders, gambling)

Assessment   **(15 %)**

14. Assessment procedures:
    a. Behavioral observations
    b. Interview
    c. Functional skills testing
    d. Current TR/leisure assessment instruments
    e. Other inventories and questionnaires
15. Assessment process:
    a. Other sources of assessment data (e.g., records, other professionals)
    b. Selection (e.g., reliability, validity, practicality, availability)
    c. Implementation
    d. Interpretation
16. Assessment domains:
    a. Sensory (e.g., vision, hearing, tactile)
    b. Cognitive (e.g., memory, problem solving, attention span, orientation, safety awareness)
    c. Social (e.g., communication/interactive skills, relationships)
    d. Physical (e.g., fitness, motor skill function)
    e. Emotional (e.g., attitude toward self, expression)
    f. Leisure (e.g., barriers, interests, attitudes, patterns/skills, knowledge)

Planning the Intervention   **(15%)**

17. Program issues related to impairments:
    a. Impact of impairment on the person served
    b. Normalization and inclusion and least restrictive environment
    c. Architectural barriers and accessibility
    d. Societal attitudes (e.g., stereotypes)
    e. Legislation (Americans with Disabilities Act, Individuals with Disabilities Act, Older Americans Act, New Freedom Initiative)
18. Standards of practice for the TR Profession
19. Code of ethics in the TR field and accepted ethical practices with respect to cultural, social, spiritual, and ethnic differences
20. Nature and diversity of recreation and leisure activities
21. Purpose and techniques of activity analysis
22. Relevant guidelines and standards (e.g., federal and state regulatory agencies, accrediting agencies, payment systems)
23. Leisure education (e.g., knowledge, resources, skills)
24. Selection of programs and interventions to achieve the assessed needs of the person served
25. Assistive techniques, technology, and adaptive devices
26. Methods of writing measurable goals and behavioral objectives
27. Role and function of other health and human service professionals and of interdisciplinary approaches
28. Use of quality improvement guidelines in program planning and implementation

**Implementing the Individualized
Intervention Plan**   **(16%)**

29. Principles of group interaction and leadership
30. Principles of behavioral change (e.g., self-efficacy theory, experiential learning model)
31. Related intervention techniques:
    a. Behavior management techniques (e.g., behavior modification, self-regulation, coping skills)
    b. Stress management (e.g., relaxation techniques)
    c. Assertiveness training
    d. Remotivation

    e. Reality orientation
    f. Cognitive retraining
    g. Counseling techniques
    h. Sensory stimulation
    i. Methods for educating and incorporating families and relevant others
    j. Validation and values clarification
    k. Social skills training

Documentation and Evaluation   **(15%)**

32. Methods of documenting assessment, progress/functional status, discharge/transition plan of the person served
33. Documentation procedures for program accountability, and payment for services
34. Methods for interpretation of progress notes, observations, and assessment results of the person served.
35. Methods for evaluating agency/TR service program
36. Methods for quality improvement

Organizing and Managing Services   **(9 %)**

37. Components of agency/TR Service plan of operation
38. Personnel, intern, and volunteer supervision and management
39. Budgeting and fiscal responsibility for service delivery
40. Area and facility management
41. Quality improvement (e.g., utilization review, risk management, peer review, outcome monitoring)
42. Payment systems (e.g., managed care, PPO, private contract, Medicare, Medicaid)
43. Accreditation standards and regulations (e.g., JCAHO, CARF, CMS)

Advancement of the Profession   **(7 %)**

44. Professionalism: Guidelines for the development of the profession
45. Requirements for TR certification/recertification
46. Advocacy for persons served
47. Legislation and regulations pertaining to TR (Healthy People, 2010)
48. Professional standards and ethical guidelines pertaining to TR

49. Public relations, promotion and marketing of the TR profession
50. Methods, resources and references for maintaining and upgrading professional competencies
51. Knowledge of professional associations and organizations
52. Interactive process among pre-services, in-service, and direct service for the advancement of the TR profession (e.g., internships, collaborative research, presentations)

* The Required Knowledge Areas from the NCTRC website was the basis of this table although the numbering was changed to basic outlining to make it more understandable for this chapter. (www.NCTRC.org retrieved April 2004.)

Background

Approximately eight percent of the exam was derived from the knowledge area *Background*. This translates into approximately seven questions. This knowledge area is to ensure that the entry-level professional has an understanding of the theoretical and conceptual basis of therapeutic recreation. Background begins with the competencies of growth and development, human behavior change, diversity factors and then proceeds into some general subtopics consisting of Leisure: Theories and Concepts, Therapeutic Recreation, and Service Delivery Systems, each of which has competencies.

Understanding *human growth and development* is an important aspect of therapeutic recreation. Having a general understanding of a person's general growth and development (cognitive, physical, emotional, and social) helps to establish realistic expectations of clients and provide appropriate interventions and treatment plans. The following material is very generic and does not try to cover all the changes that occur during a life stage.

Early childhood consists of those ages between birth and around six. During this time a child should be developing fundamental motor skills and social skills; a child's body is changing rapidly, and most children are very interested in finding out what exactly their limits are cognitively, physically, socially, and emotionally. Communication skills are also developing. Play is very important for children of these ages, for it is through play that many of their skills are developed and enhanced.

Children are those between the ages of six and 12. During this time the child's social world expands; he or she begins to be involved in organized sports and games and extracurricular activities such as dance classes and music lessons. Children are still very involved in play, and their hand/eye coordination is improving. As the child grows older, friends become more significant than family and being like everyone else becomes very important.

Adolescence is the next stage and covers the ages between 13 and 21, approximately. This is the time when peer groups (peer pressure) become more important than family, and an individual struggles to become more independent from the family. The body begins to reach maturation and the interest in intimate relationships increases. Sexuality becomes intense with hormones influencing behavior. Organized sports, music, and the "mall" become very important. Individuals are usually beginning to define themselves in their own right (e.g., as athletes or perhaps scholars). Peer groups continue to be important, but by the end of older adolescence, family is regaining its importance.

Individuals in the early adulthood stages (ages 21–30) usually establish their independence by completing their education and seeking their own occupation. During this time, they may begin to have more serious intimate relationships in order to establish families of their own. Their bodies have reached maturation, and the interest may be on more challenging leisure activities such as rock climbing or other activities that allow for the growth of relationships, such as movies and dinners. This is also the time when a person may develop an interest in more life-long leisure pursuits, such as golf, tennis, or running.

The years between 30 and 45 are known as middle adulthood. A person's family and career take priority. During this period many adults find themselves actively involved in their childrens' leisure pursuits. They attend sporting activities, concerts, plays, etc., and volunteer as coaches and leaders for various youth organizations. Their activities are very family oriented, such as game nights, family vacations, etc. Occasionally, the individual is involved in individual pursuits such as golf or running.

Older adulthood occurs approximately between the ages of 45 and 60. For most people there is a slowing down, and as the metabolism begins to change, there is a weight gain. Physical abilities also change with reductions in strength and flexibility. Cognitively, however, skills and abilities remain strong. This is the life stage where people may experience midlife crises and depression. Children have moved out and the parents of people in this life stage are becoming dependent. It can be a very stressful time in life, yet it can also be very freeing when parents are still healthy and their own children are having children and advancing in their own careers.

Senior adulthood is the stage between 60 and 75. Most people have great amounts of free time and are retired. Although many individuals are beginning to experience health problems, most individuals are healthy, vigorous, and have the freedom to travel and participate in activities of their choosing.

The "old-old" stage occurs from age 75 to death. For some people, physical deterioration is rapid, and for others it is cognitive deterioration that seems to occur rapidly. All people

in this age group will experience health problems and need assistance. Their world may become smaller due to the death of friends and the need to live in a facility that can provide the assistance they need. Although many people will be limited in their abilities, there are others who will continue to be active (Edgington, Jordan, DeGraf, & Edgington, 2002; Feil, 1993; Godbey, 2003; Jordan, 2001; Russell, 2001).

It is assumed that entry-level professionals will understand *theories of human behavior change*, which includes self-efficacy, the attribution model, and the concept of learned helplessness. The entry-level professional needs to understand not only the concepts, but also how clients/patients might display these behaviors. When a person displays self-efficacy, essentially he or she is demonstrating the expectations of his or her ability to cope with his or her problems. A person must be confident of his abilities and not give up when the results of his or her actions are not immediate. If a person has recently become a paraplegic and is able to begin thinking of changes in his leisure activities (i.e., the adaptations necessary, trying them out, and not giving up when the results are not perfect), the person is beginning to cope and probably has good self-efficacy.

The attribution model deals with a person's explanation of the cause of events that occurred in that person's life. A person may explain the event due to internal or external attributes. For example, a client might believe that he was fired due to the "boss's dislike of him," which is an "external attribute," rather than his not completing tasks on time, which would be an "internal attribute." Understanding what attributes the client assigns to events will help the therapist work with the client. Helping the client to understand his role in an event is very important for the client's growth.

Learned helplessness is another theory of behavior change that the entry-level professional needs to understand. According to Mannell and Kleiber (1997), learned helplessness is "the phenomenon in which experience with uncontrollable events creates passive behavior toward subsequent threats to well being" (p. 134). For example, when a client experiences consistent failure in physical activities as a child, she may refuse to try new physical activities as an adult because of that early failure, or she may try them but put little effort in achieving success because of her belief that she will not succeed (Austin, 2004; Iso-Ahola, 1980; Mannell & Kleiber, 1997; Shank & Coyle, 2002).

In many ways the United States is becoming a more *diverse* nation. With this *diversity,* we recognize that many cultures and socioeconomic groups make up our country. As a result there are "pockets" of cultural differences in relation to beliefs about recreation, leisure, and disability. It is important that the entry-level therapist understands and respects those differences. Thus, along with understanding the impact of various life stages, it is important to have an understanding of the impact of diversity. According to Getz (2002), "Knowledge of the patient's cultural background can...ultimately increase the overall success of the treatment process."

Besides basic competencies, this knowledge area is divided into three subtopics: recreation, leisure, and play; therapeutic recreation; and service delivery systems. Competencies are then identified under these subtopics.

The subtopic of *leisure* has several competencies under it. It is believed that all entry-level professionals should have a basic understanding of *leisure theories and concepts.* As a professional who will teach patients/clients about leisure, the entry-level professional must have an understanding of how people view leisure. The entry-level professional must understand the difference between leisure as time, leisure as activity, leisure as a state of mind, leisure as a symbol of social status, leisure as an anti-utilitarian concept, and leisure as a holistic concept. When working with a client who, when asked, says "leisure is skiing," the therapeutic recreation specialist understands that the client believes that leisure is activity, and so has a starting point for leisure education. Thus, it is very important that the entry-level professional understands the differing views of leisure (Edgington, Jordan, DeGraf & Edgington 2002; Godbey 2003; Russell 2001).

Building upon this basic knowledge is an understanding of some basic *social psychology aspects in relation to leisure* that include perceived freedom, intrinsic motivation and locus of control. Perceived freedom implies that people think they have a choice, and in this instance it is used in relation to leisure. According to most leisure professionals, people do not really have leisure unless they at least believe they have the freedom to choose what they do during their leisure. Intrinsic motivation is another concept used in relation to leisure. People must be motivated from within to have a truly leisure experience; external factors (i.e., other people, money, etc.) cannot be the motivating reason. Locus of control relates to the amount of control a person feels he has over the events that occur in his life. If a person believes that for the most part he controls the outcome of events, he is said to have "internal locus of control." If a person believes that the outcome of events is largely "due to luck, the environment or others," then he is said to have "external locus of control" (Austin 2004; Edgington, Jordan, DeGraaf, & Edgington, 2002; Iso-Ahola, 1980; Mannell & Kleiber, 1997; Neulinger, 1974).

Leisure throughout the lifespan is another competency. Although there are not specific activities that one must participate in during a specific life stage within his lifespan, one can identify general activities that one might participate in dependent upon his life stage. For example, a single person in his or her 20s is more likely to go backpacking in the mountains alone than a married person in his or her 40s. Understanding a person's life stage will help the entry-level therapist develop a program that will meet patient's interests and needs. Some of the information for this competency may be found under the *Human Growth and Development* competency (Edginton, Jordan, DeGraff, & Edginton, 2002).

Leisure lifestyle development is another important competency for the entry-level therapeutic recreation specialist. Leisure can influence lifestyle. According to Edginton, Jordan, DeGraff, and Edginton (2002), "The work of a leisure services professional, along with encouraging life satisfaction, should focus on facilitating both social (behavioral) and environmental (physical) conditions that help people achieve optimal lifestyles" (p. 13). Leisure can assist the individual in developing a healthy, satisfying lifestyle (Edginton, Jordan, DeGraff, & Edginton, 2002).

The second subtopic is *therapeutic recreation*. The first competency in this subtopic is *concepts of therapeutic recreation*. One needs to have a thorough understanding of therapeutic recreation in general. To understand therapeutic recreation, one must believe in the treatment of the "whole person." This approach to therapeutic recreation fits into the holistic health model. So when a woman is referred to therapeutic recreation due to a stroke, the therapist is concerned not only with the patient's physical and cognitive well being but also her emotional, social, and spiritual well being. The therapist is concerned with the patient's deficits and her strengths and what changes might help her when she goes home and assist in the prevention of another stroke.

An understanding of the value of the recreative experience is also important for the therapeutic recreation specialist to understand and appreciate. For all people, recreation experiences can provide relaxation, they can stimulate the mind, allow adventure, enable socialization, etc. Clients need to learn the impact that their choices of recreation experiences can have on their quality of life (Carter, van Andel, & Robb, 2003; Kraus & Shank, 1992).

Also within the subtopic of *Therapeutic Recreation* is a competency related to *models of service delivery*. A variety of models is listed within this competency. According to Kraus and Shank (1992), special recreation is the provision of programs and opportunities for individuals with disabilities to develop, maintain, and express a self-directed, personally satisfying lifestyle that actively involves leisure (p. 34). Recreation for persons with disabilities in the community, Special Olympics, or wheelchair basketball tournaments are examples of this model with which the entry-level professional is expected to be familiar.

The Leisure Ability, or Therapeutic Recreation Service Model, seems to be the most widely accepted and utilized model and is composed of the following three components: functional intervention, leisure education, and recreation participation. According to Stumbo and Peterson (2004), "The ultimate goal [of the Leisure Ability Model]. . .is a satisfying leisure lifestyle—the independent functioning of the client in leisure experiences and activities of his or her choice" (pp. 38-39). The therapist assesses the client's need, provides the necessary functional intervention, leisure education, and recreation participation services, and evaluates the degree to which the client met the desired outcomes.

The Health Protection/Health Promotion Model can be seen as having two components: a) helping a patient recover from threats to health (health protection); and b) helping a client achieve optimal health (health promotion) through the use of prescriptive activities, recreation, and leisure. Austin (2002) states that the "mission of therapeutic recreation is to assist persons to move toward an optimal state of health" (p. 9). There are four basic underlying concepts of the health protection/health promotion model. They are: a humanistic perspective, high-level wellness, the stabilization and actualization tendencies, and health.

The Service Delivery Model provides what its author considers the scope of services involved in therapeutic recreation. Its four components include: 1) Diagnosis/Needs Assessment, 2) Treatment/Rehabilitation of a problem or need, 3) Educational Services, and 4) Prevention/Health Promotion activities. "The model is intended to represent a continuum of service delivery—from the more intense, acute-care approach involving diagnosis and treatment found in hospitals or rehabilitation centers to the community-based focus on outpatient, day treatment, or home health care services that generally emphasize education and health promotion activities" (Carter, van Andel, & Robb, 2004, p. 23). The Therapeutic Recreation Outcome Model is an extension of the Service Delivery Model. This model looks at the products (outcomes) of the delivery of therapeutic recreation services. It takes into account changes in functional capacities and health status which, according to the model, will ultimately impact quality of life.

The activity therapy model is one of the oldest models and is used primarily in psychiatric hospitals. This model proposes a variety of "action" therapies, including recreation therapy, music therapy, art therapy, dance therapy, and occupational therapy. All provide programs for clients and are usually housed in the same department—"Activity Therapy." Any therapist from this department could be utilized to provide programming for clients dependent on the program desired.

Many hospitals are utilizing the "treatment model" which instead of writing goals and treatment plans by specialized area (i.e., recreation therapy, physical therapy, and occupational therapy, etc.), goals are determined by treatment teams, and each therapist works on the same treatment goals utilizing his unique area of expertise (Austin, 2002; Carter, van Andel & Robb, 2003; Dattilo, 2002; Kennedy, Austin, & Smith, 2001; Kraus & Shank, 1992; Mosey, 1973; Ross & Ashton-Schaeffer, 2001; Stumbo, 2001; Stumbo & Peterson, 2004).

The *historical development of therapeutic recreation* is a competency found in this section. The use of activities as a therapeutic tool can be traced back to the beginning of civilization. However, its history in the U.S. probably began with the development of some of the specialty schools, institutions, or hospitals for persons with visual impairments, physical disabilities, emotional disorders or developmental disabilities (Carter, van Andel & Robb, 2003). Its roots can also be found with the rise of the playground movement, which was used to prevent delinquency. Therapeutic recreation continued its sporadic growth until WWI when the American Red Cross used recreational activities to treat those who sustained various injuries in military combat. The Red Cross continued to employ and train recreation leaders during WWII. In the 1930s the Menninger Clinic, following the psychoanalytic model of treatment of psychiatric disorders, used activities to help clients learn to reduce tension, anxiety, and release aggression appropriately. In the 1950s Beatrice Hill established

"Comeback, Inc.," which promoted recreation services in the community for non-institutionalized people with disabilities and also promoted recreation for persons who were hospitalized or in a special school or nursing home. Also during this time period, Janet Pomeroy founded the San Francisco Recreation Center for the Handicapped. During the 1950s and 1960s, community-based recreation programs for people with disabilities continued to grow. In the 1980s, health care began to go through major changes in order to contain costs. Hospitals needed to be accountable for the quality, appropriateness, and outcome of their services.

Although the above is a very brief history of therapeutic recreation, more information can be found in most introductory textbooks.

The history of the profession is probably more succinctly written by date as follows:

- 1949—Hospital Recreation Section (HRS) of the American Recreation Society was formed comprised of primarily hospital recreation workers from military, veterans, and public institutions who emphasized leisure experiences for hospitalized individuals.
- 1952—The Recreation Therapy Section (RTS) within the Recreation Section of the American Association of Health, Physical Education and Recreation was formed by people primarily with a physical education background who offered recreation and physical education programs in schools that served people with disabilities.
- 1953—The National Association of Recreational Therapists (NART) formed to serve the needs of the people who were recreational therapists in state hospitals or schools serving people with mental illness or mental retardation.
- 1953—Representatives of each organization formed the Council for the

Advancement of Hospital Recreation (CAHR) to address common problems.
- 1956—CAHR established the first voluntary registration plan for hospital recreation.
- October 1966—The HRS and NART merged to form the National Therapeutic Recreation Society, a branch of the National Recreation and Park Association. Thus, NTRS also became responsible for administration of the voluntary registration plan.
- 1981—The NTRS Registration Board separated from NTRS/NRPA and became an independent certifying body for the therapeutic recreation profession: the National Council for Therapeutic Recreation Certification (NCTRC).
- 1984—The American Therapeutic Recreation Association was established.

Because the above outline does not go into depth, the reader is encouraged to read entry-level texts and gain an understanding of how and why these organizations came into existence (Carter, van Andel, & Robb, 2003; Kraus & Shank, 1992).

Practice settings are also found within the subtopic of *Therapeutic Recreation*. An entry-level professional needs to understand how therapeutic recreation is practiced in a variety of settings, (e.g., community recreation, physical rehabilitation centers, psychiatric hospitals, out patient clinics, day treatment programs, long-term care facilities, etc.). However, it is important to keep in mind that the process of therapeutic recreation—assess, plan, implement, and evaluate—is constant, no matter where therapeutic recreation is being practiced. Therapeutic recreation is a "process" and is not "setting dependent."

Another subtopic is *Service Delivery Systems*. One of the competencies covered within this subtopic is *health care*. The majority of therapeutic recreation services are found in a health care facility, be it a rehabilitation hospital, a community hospital, an outpatient unit, or a pediatric unit, all are found in the health care service delivery system. It is important to understand what makes this service delivery "health care." Is it how the services are offered? The types of services offered? Usually in health care services, treatment is prescribed by either the physician or the treatment team. When therapeutic recreation is prescribed, the therapeutic recreation process (assess, plan, implement, and evaluate) becomes activated and specific programs and interventions are determined based on the assessment.

Leisure services are another service delivery system. Usually the client is referred either through self-referral or by another therapeutic recreation specialist as part of the client's discharge plan from health care. Leisure services are usually community based and may be segregated or the client may be participating in inclusive recreation. If the services are segregated, the therapeutic recreation specialist will follow the same therapeutic recreation process to determine the most appropriate program for the client. If the services are inclusive, then the client chooses what recreation/leisure service they would like to be involved in (Carter & LeConey, 2004; Carter, van Andel, & Robb, 2003; Kennedy, Austin, & Smith, 2001; Kennedy & Montgomery, 1998; Shank & Coyle, 2002).

Education services are the last service delivery system. Due to the inclusion of recreation as a related service in the Individuals with Disabilities Education Act, therapeutic recreation specialists can be found in the school system, specifically in special education services. All students eligible for special education services must have an individualized education plan (IEP). The IEP outlines the services that are necessary for the student to achieve his goals and objectives and the IEP can specify therapeutic recreation services. Within the IEP, depending on the age of the child, there may be a section labeled "transition." The Individualized Transition Plan projects "post school" goals and methods to ensure those goals will become reality. This section may specifically address leisure goals and objectives. The therapeutic recreation specialist may assist in the development of the goals and objectives but will certainly provide the necessary programming to meet those goals and objectives, once again utilizing the therapeutic recreation process (Bullock & Johnson, 1998; Bullock & Mahon, 2001; Lawson, Coyle, & Ashton-Shaeffer, 2001).

The last competency in *Background* is *models of health care and human services.* As an entry-level professional, you need to have an understanding of the medical model, since many hospitals utilize this model. Also the psychosocial rehabilitation model is used in many health-care facilities. Health and wellness have grown and become a function of many health care facilities. Thus, you need to have a basic understanding of these models. The person-centered model seems to be the model that is used by therapeutic recreation personnel in all areas of service.

The content that is covered in this first knowledge area, *Background*, is usually taught in introductory recreation/leisure courses and in introductory therapeutic recreation courses. The social psychology concepts are covered in some introductory leisure texts and some therapeutic recreation texts. The human growth and development material is contained in most human growth and development courses and often can be found in leadership and programming courses. Leisure, recreation, and play concepts are found in introductory leisure and recreation texts. Most introductory texts and courses in therapeutic recreation adequately cover the material in the subtopics of Therapeutic Recreation and Service Delivery Systems.

References Related to Background

Allison, M. T., & Schneider, I. E. (Eds.). (2000). *Diversity and the recreation profession: Organizational perspectives.* State College, PA: Venture Publishing.

Austin, D. R. (2004). *Therapeutic recreation: Processes and techniques* (5th ed.). Champaign, IL: Sagamore Publishing.

Austin, D. R. (2002). Conceptual models in therapeutic recreation. In D. R. Austin, J. Dattilo, & B. P. McCormick (Eds.), *Conceptual foundations in therapeutic recreation* (pp.1-27). State College, PA: Venture Publishing, Inc.

Bullock, C. C., & Johnson, D. E. (1998). *Recreation therapy in special education.* In F. Brasile, T. K. Skalko, & J. Burlingame (Eds.), *Perspectives in recreation therapy: Issues of a dynamic profession* (pp. 107-124). Ravensdale, WA: Idyll Arbor.

Bullock, C. C., & Mahon, M. J. (2001). *Introduction to recreation services for people with disabilities: A person-centered approach* (2nd ed.). Champaign, IL: Sagamore Publishing.

Carter, M. J., & LeConey, S. P., (2004). *Therapeutic recreation in the community: An inclusive approach* (2nd ed.). Champaign, IL: Sagamore Publishing.

Carter, M. J., Van Andel, G. E., & Robb, G. M. (2003). *Therapeutic recreation: A practical approach* (3rd ed.). Prospect Heights, IL: Waveland Press.

Dattilo, J. (2002). *Inclusive leisure services: Responding to the rights of people with disabilities* (2nd ed.). State College, PA: Venture Publishing.

Edginton, C. R., Jordan, D. J., DeGraaf, D. G., & Edginton, S. R. (2002). *Leisure and life satisfaction: Foundational perspectives* (3rd ed.). Boston, MA: McGraw Hill.

Feil, N. (1993). *The validation breakthrough.* Baltimore, MD: Health Professions Press.

Getz, D. (2002). Increasing cultural competence in therapeutic recreation. In D. R. Austin, J. Dattilo, & B. P. McCormick (Eds.), *Conceptual foundations in therapeutic recreation* (pp. 151-163). State College, PA: Venture Publishing.

Godbey, G. (2003). *Leisure in your life: An exploration.* State College, PA: Venture Publishing.

Iso-Ahola, S. E. (1980). *The social psychology of leisure and recreation.* Dubuque, IA: Wm. C. Brown.

Jordan, D. J. (2001). *Leadership in leisure services: Making a difference.* State College, PA: Venture Publishing.

Kennedy, D. W., Austin, D. R., & Smith, R. W. (2001). *Special recreation: Opportunities for people with disabilities* (4th ed.). Dubuque, IA: Wm C. Brown & Co.

Kennedy, B. S., & Montgomery, N. D. (1998). Recreation therapy in the community. In F. Brasile, T. K. Skalko, & J. Burlingame (Eds.), *Perspectives in recreation therapy: Issues of a dynamic profession* (pp. 125-140). Ravensdale, WA: Idyll Arbor.

Kraus, R., & Shank, J. (1992). *Therapeutic recreation service: Principles and practices* (4th ed.). Dubuque, IA: Brown Publishing.

Lawson, L. M., Coyle, C. P., & Ashton-Shaeffer, C. (2001). *Therapeutic recreation in special education: An IDEA for the future.* Alexandria, VA: American Therapeutic Recreation Association.

Mannell, R. C., & Kleiber, D. (1997). *A social psychology of leisure.* State College, PA: Venture Publishing.

Mosey, A. C. (1973). *Activities therapy.* New York, NY: Raven Press.

Neulinger, J. (1974). *The psychology of leisure.* Springfield, IL: Charles C. Thomas.

Ross, J. E., & Ashton-Shaeffer, C. (2001). Therapeutic recreation practice models. In N. J. Stumbo (Ed.), *Professional issues in therapeutic recreation: On competence and outcomes* (pp. 159-187). Champaign, IL: Sagamore Publishing.

Russell, R. V. (2001). *Leadership in recreation* (2nd ed.). Boston, MA: McGraw Hill.

Shank, J., & Coyle, C. (2002). *Therapeutic recreation in health promotion and rehabilitation.* State College, PA: Venture Publishing.

Stumbo, N. (2001). *Professional issues in therapeutic recreation: On competence and outcomes.* Champaign, IL: Sagamore Publishing.

Stumbo, N. J., & Peterson, C. A. (2004). *Therapeutic recreation program design: Principles and procedures* (4th ed.). San Francisco, CA: Benjamin Cummings.

Sylvester, C., Voelkl, J. E., & Ellis, G. D. (2001). *Therapeutic recreation programming: Theory and practice.* State College, PA: Venture Publishing.

Diagnostic Groupings and Populations Served

From the knowledge area *Diagnostic Groupings and Populations Served,* approximately 15 percent or 13 questions will be derived. This knowledge area is to ensure that the entry-level professional has an understanding of people with disabilities and the effects of their disabling conditions on their lives. The competencies within this area are Cognitive Impairments, Physical Impairments, Sensory and Communication Impairments, Psychiatric Impairments, Behavioral Impairments, and Addictions. These subtopics encompass the disabling conditions that affect the people with whom therapeutic recreation professionals work.

The first competency is *Cognitive Impairments.* Within this subtopic, all disabling conditions that have an impact on a person's cognitive abilities are addressed. One of the primary populations within this subtopic is persons with developmental disabilities. When developmental disabilities were first mentioned in legislation (the Developmental Disabilities Assistance Bill of Rights Act of 1970) specific types of disabilities (mental retardation, cerebral palsy, epilepsy) were classified as developmental disabilities. However, when the law was reenacted (the Rehabilitation Comprehensive Services, and Developmental Disabilities Amendments of 1978) a more functional definition was substituted (Carter, van Andel, & Robb, 2003; Mobily & MacNeil, 2002).

A developmental disability is "a severe and chronic disorder involving mental and/or physical impairment that originates before age 22. Such a disorder is likely to persist indefinitely and cause substantial functional limitations in at least three of seven areas of major life activity, including self-care, receptive and expressive language, learning, mobility, self-direction, capacity for independent living, and economic self-sufficiency" (Mobily & MacNeil, 2002, p. 15).

Most people who are mentally retarded are developmentally disabled. A person who is classified as mentally retarded has scored significantly (a minimum of two standard deviations) below average on a standardized IQ test. The most commonly used classification system is the one used by the American Psychiatric Association (2000): mild, moderate, severe, and profound. Entry-level professionals need to know what these levels of mental retardation mean in regards to the functioning of the individual, any special teaching/learning characteristics that are necessary dependent on functioning level and any activity protocols that have been developed for this population.

Most individuals with autism have functional characteristics that enable them to be classified as developmentally disabled. Autism is considered to be a spectrum disorder because the symptoms and characteristics present themselves in a wide variety of combinations. Behavioral symptoms can range from hyperactivity, short attention span, impulsivity, to self-injurious behaviors. An individual can have problems with sensory stimulation (oversensitivity to sound or touch), eating, sleeping, and an absence of emotional reaction (i.e., no reaction to pain) or excessive fear. There may also be a problem with speech (echolalia), poor eye contact, resistance to change, and sustained odd play. Entry-level professionals need to have a basic understanding of the symptoms of autism, its prognosis, and treatment. You also need to have a basic understanding about the unique needs of a person with autism in regard to the environment and leadership techniques.

Also included in *Cognitive Impairments* are persons with traumatic brain injury (TBI). Persons with TBI have generally been involved in an accident and may have other complications that involve their physical abilities. It is important to understand the different levels of brain injury; thus, one needs to know/understand both the Glasgow Coma Scale and the Rancho Los Amigos Scale. Also, one needs to have a basic understanding of the brain so if an injury occurred in a specific area of the brain, one would generally know what the cognitive effects might be. In addition, one needs to be familiar with the treatment of persons with brain injury, the value of recreation therapy in treatment, and any specific protocols used with this population. It is also important to be aware of the effect of having a brain-injured person in the family.

A group of people who experience effects similar to persons with traumatic brain injury are those who have had a cardiovascular accident (CVA) or stroke that is essentially an interruption of the blood-flow to the brain. Strokes may be caused by a cerebral thrombosis, hemorrhage, or embolism. Hemiplegia is a sign of a stroke. Damage to the right side of the brain may cause left hemiplegia, problems with depth perception, visual neglect, problems orienting to the environment and estimating abilities. Damage to the left side of the brain will cause right hemiplegia, and individuals may have problems speaking (aphasia), understanding, reading, writing and judgment. They may also have problems with new situations. It is important to understand the impact of a CVA on a person, the general protocol one might use to treat a person who has had a CVA, and, again, the impact on family life.

Dementia is also considered a *Cognitive Impairment.* There are a variety of types of dementia including Alzheimer's Disease, Vascular Dementia, Dementia with Lewy Bodies, Pick's Disease, Parkinson's disease, Alcohol-related dementia, and Wernicke-Korsakoff Syndrome. According to Buettner and Fitzsimmons (2003), there are two sets of symptoms that an entry-level therapeutic recreation specialist needs to be aware of: behavioral symptoms and cognitive symptoms. Although the loss of cognitive skills and memory is disturbing, it is the behavioral symptoms (apathy, physical aggression or nonaggression, verbal nonaggression or aggression, or refusal of care, medication, etc.) that cause the most difficulty for caregivers. Persons with dementia may also experience depression, paranoia, social withdrawal or suicidal ideation (pp. 11-12). The most common form of dementia is Alzheimer's Disease (AD). There are three stages of AD: Stage One or Mild lasts between two and four years, Stage Two or Moderate lasts from two to seven years, and the Third Stage is Severe and lasts from one to three years. Each stage is distinctive and has its own symptoms. The entry-level therapeutic recreation specialist needs to be aware of and understand the protocols that have been developed for the care of persons with dementia.

"Epilepsy is a chronic brain disorder characterized by recurring attacks of abnormal sensory, motor, and psychological activity" (Tamparo & Lewis, 2000, p. 235). A seizure disorder is a common neurological condition that can be either primary or secondary epilepsy. If a seizure has no identifiable etiology, then it can be classified as "primary." If it occurs after an impact to the brain and seizures occur, it would be classified as a "secondary" condition. A "partial" seizure involves only one cerebral hemisphere, while a "generalized" seizure involves both hemispheres. Seizures may also be classified as "simple," no loss of consciousness, or "complex" in which a person loses consciousness (American Psychiatric Association, 2000; Bender & Baglin, 2004; Buettner & Fitzsimmons, 2003; Carter & LeConey, 2004; Carter, van Andel, & Robb, 2003; Coyne & Fullerton, 2004; Mobily & MacNeil, 2002; Tamparo & Lewis, 2000; Wilhite & Keller, 2000).

Physical Impairment seems to be the largest competency in the *Diagnostic Groupings and Populations Served* Knowledge Area. It seems almost any impairment that does not fit under cognitive, sensory, or psychiatric is considered to be physical, thus this category ranges from a total hip replacement to AIDS. These impairments may cause an adjustment in a person's activities for a period of time but may not cause a complete change of lifestyle. It is important to understand the treatment of these disorders and the type of adapted equipment that the person may temporarily or permanently require.

Cerebral Palsy (CP) is a developmental disorder that is characterized by problems controlling movement. It is a non-progressive disorder. CP can be classified by limb involvement (quadriplegia, paraplegia, diplegia, hemiplegia, triplegia, or monoplegia) or by exhibited symptoms (spasticity, athetosis, or ataxia). As an entry-level therapeutic recreation specialist, you need to understand the functional characteristics of the classifications mentioned. As an entry-level therapeutic recreation specialist, you need to understand the impact of CP on the individual and their needs. Primarily, therapeutic recreation specialists will work with individuals with CP in community settings.

Muscular Dystrophy (MD) is a group of related diseases that affect the musculoskeletal system. Duchenne or childhood muscular dystrophy is the most severe and common form of MD. It affects male children who begin to show symptoms by the age of two or three. This is a progressive disease. By adolescence, most persons who have Duchenne use a wheelchair and by adulthood usually are confined to a bed. Most men with Duchenne die in their early 20s. There are two other types of MD that affect adults: facio-scapulo-humeral and limb-girdle. These types affect both males and females. It is important to understand the effects of MD on the person's leisure, help them make necessary adaptations, and, as the MD progresses, help the person and the families deal with the changes.

Spinal cord injury includes persons who have paraplegia or quadriplegia. Spinal cord injuries are usually acquired through trauma. The level of injury is identified by the initial area of the spinal cord where the lesion occurs. A person whose cord is severed above the second thoracic vertebra (T2) has quadriplegia, and a person who has an injury at or below the second thoracic vertebra has paraplegia. Also the lesion can be labeled complete or incomplete. Thus, it is important for the entry-level therapeutic recreation specialist to understand the effects of the location of the lesion and what it means when a lesion is complete or incomplete on a person's functioning level. The therapeutic recreation specialist is expected to help the individual use his residual skills to regain as much independence as possible and to assist in the treatment of secondary conditions such as depression or adjustment to disability. It is important to understand the treatment protocols for persons with spinal cord injury, the benefits of therapeutic recreation, and equipment adaptations. Community reintegration is an important treatment component for persons who are coping with spinal cord injury.

Multiple Sclerosis (MS) is a disease that impacts the nervous system. It is commonly diagnosed in individuals who are between the ages of 20 and 50. MS causes deterioration of the myelin sheath. There is no set pattern of symptoms, but commonly a person has speech disturbances, balance problems, vertigo, blurred vision, walking difficulties, and tremors. There is a pattern of exacerbation and remission, but there is never a complete recovery to the original functioning level. An entry-level professional must understand the progression of this disorder, its prognosis, and treatment of this condition. It is important to understand the impact of this disorder on a person's life and the adjustments to be made in their lifestyle.

Diseases of the circulatory system are also included under *Physical Impairments*. A thera-peutic recreation specialist may work with persons who are recovering from a myocardial infarction or have specific heart conditions that may impact their treatment. The American Heart Association has established functional ability limitations ranging from Class I (no limitation of physical activity) to Class IV (inability to carry on any physical activity without discomfort). The therapeutic recreation specialist must understand the prognosis of these diseases, restrictions, and assist the person in the development of a healthy lifestyle.

Also within *Physical Impairments* are diseases of the endocrine and metabolic systems. This includes persons learning to cope with diabetes mellitus. A person who is diagnosed with diabetes has large amounts of sugar in the blood and urine. Immune-mediated diabetes type 1 usually is diagnosed before age 30. It is usually very difficult to regulate and the person is usually on insulin. Type 2 diabetes is more common and appears in adults older than 40. This form of diabetes can be managed by diet, but some people may require insulin. Entry-level professionals may need to know how to assist people in coping with their diabetes and the impact of exercise on their insulin levels.

Infectious diseases are also included within *Physical Impairments*. Entry-level professionals need to have an understanding of a variety of cancers, their prognosis, and treatment. Cancer includes a group of more than 100 diseases. A tumor may be benign or malignant. If it is malignant, a tumor is invasive, grows rapidly and can metastasize through the circulatory or lymph system. Tumors can be graded (1-4) and staged using a TNM system: T (refers to the size and extent of the primary tumor), N (refers to the number of area lymph nodes involved), and M (refers to any metastasis of the primary tumor). Entry-level therapeutic recreation specialists need to understand the role of a therapeutic recreation specialist in assisting the person in attaining/continuing quality of life. Therapeutic recreation specialists can address the psychosocial impact of cancer.

Autoimmune Deficiency Syndrome (AIDS) is a viral infection associated with the human immunodeficiency virus (HIV). The virus is usually transmitted through sexual intercourse, but it can be transmitted by blood and blood products. AIDS produces a spectrum of symptoms. It is imperative that entry-level professionals understand the etiology of this disease, necessary precautions, prognosis, and treatment. This disease also requires that the therapeutic recreation specialist be able to help the client/patient cope with an incurable illness and continue a quality of life that is appealing to him or her.

This section has tried to present some of the major physical impairments. It is not possible or feasible to adequately cover all the potential physical impairments which an entry-level professional may be expected to understand. The clients/patients you will be working with may be in a variety of rehabilitative stages (Bender & Baglin, 2004; Carter, van Andel, & Robb, 2003; Mobily & MacNeil, 2002; Tamparo & Lewis, 2000).

Sensory and Communication Impairments is the third competency in *Diagnostic Groupings and Populations Served*. The entry-level professional needs to have an understanding of the person who is visually impaired or blind. The etiology of the impairment, how people with visual impairments learn best, and what equipment or adapted equipment is necessary to help them enjoy a satisfying leisure lifestyles are important topics. An understanding of specific leadership is also important.

Hearing impairments are also part of this competency. Again, knowing the etiology and teaching/learning techniques for persons who have hearing impairments or are deaf is important. Also an understanding of deaf culture is important. If you are going to work with persons who are deaf, it is important that you know sign language.

Speech impairments, like hearing and visual impairments may be found in all populations. It is important that you understand the different types of aphasia that may be a residual effect found with some persons who have had a CVA or another type of brain injury. Also many persons who have CP may also have problems with speech. A therapeutic recreation professional needs to demonstrate patience and listening skills when working with these individuals (Carter, van Andel, & Robb, 2003; Mobily & MacNeil, 2002).

Another competency in *Diagnostic Groupings and Populations Served* pertains to *Psychiatric Impairments*. You are expected to have a basic understanding of the treatment of a range of persons with a variety of psychiatric disorders ranging from severe psychoses to chemical dependencies to eating disorders. It is also a good idea to be familiar with the *DSM IV-TR* and its use.

It is important to have an understanding of the symptoms and treatment of persons with schizophrenia. According to the American Psychiatric Association (2000), to be diagnosed with schizophrenia, a person must have two or more of the following characteristics during a one-month period: "delusions, hallucinations, disorganized, grossly disorganized or catatonic behavior, and negative symptoms" (p. 312). It is important to understand that with schizophrenia there is always a change in functioning levels. Since schizophrenia is a group of disorders from paranoid schizophrenia to hebephrenia to catatonia, it is important to know the difference between them and the treatment protocols for these psychiatric conditions. Also, an understanding of medications and their side effects is expected. It is also important to understand the benefits of in-patient treatment and day treatment programs.

Affective disorders are those disorders that have a strong impact on emotions. They include depression and bipolar disorders. A person diagnosed with depression has a serious illness. It is not the typical day-to-day "blues." To be diagnosed with depression, a person must have five or more of the following symptoms during the same two-week period: depressed mood for most of the day, diminished interest in day-to-day activities, significant weight loss or gain, sleeplessness or sleeping all the time, psychomotor agitation, overall feeling of tiredness, feelings of worthlessness, inability to concentrate, and thoughts of suicide (American Psychiatric Association, 2000, p. 356). A person who is diagnosed with bipolar disorder not only has depression, but his moods will "swing" from the lows of depression to mania. When in a manic mode, the person will have three or more of the following symptoms: inflated self-esteem, seems not to need sleep, very talkative, highly distractible, thoughts seem to be racing, increase in goal-directed activity (feel like they can accomplish anything), and overly involved in activities that have a high possibility for a painful outcome. It is important to understand the symptoms and characteristics of these disorders, the benefits of therapeutic recreation with these populations, and potential treatment protocols. Medications can be used to help people with these impairments, and the therapeutic recreation specialist needs to be aware of the side effects of the medication.

Personality disorders are also included within this subtopic. The American Psychiatric Association lists 10 different personality disorders, clustering them together into three different categories based on descriptive similarities. Cluster A consists of paranoid, schizoid, and schizotypal personality disorders. In general, people with these personality disorders often appear odd or eccentric. Cluster B consists of the antisocial, borderline, histrionic, and narcissistic personality disorders, and these people have a commonality of being dramatic, emotional, or erratic. Cluster C consists of avoidant, dependent, and obsessive-compulsive personality disorders. The commonality between these personality disorders is anxiousness or fearfulness (American Psychiatric Association, 2000, pp. 685-686). You should be familiar with the major types and their symptoms, as well as techniques in working with this diagnostic group and any treatment protocols that have been developed.

Eating disorders are also in this diagnostic group. Unfortunately, eating disorders have become common in our society due to the emphasis on external beauty. Generally speaking, anorexia nervosa may be diagnosed when a person places himself or herself on a diet and exercise program that eventually causes starvation. An individual who has bulimia nervosa goes through a cycle of overeating and then vomiting or using laxatives (binge-purge). You need to understand the difference between anorexia nervosa and bulimia nervosa, their symptoms, prognosis, and treatment. It is a good idea to understand their functional characteristics, focusing on emotional issues and self-image. Because this disorder is thought to have a direct relationship with the family system, it is important to understand family interactions.

Although polysubstance dependence and alcohol dependence are listed under this subcategory, they are also listed under the subcategory of *Addictions* and will be addressed there (American Psychiatric Association, 2000; Baglin, Lewis, & Williams, 2004; Carter, van Andel, & Robb, 2003; Mobily & MacNeil, 2002).

Behavioral impairments make up another competency. Within this category are victims and/or perpetrators of violence, abuses or neglect. Child abuse and neglect have become a nationwide concern. According to Carter, van Andel, and Robb (2003), "Abuse is an act of commission or inflicting injury or allowing injury to a child, while neglect refers to an act of omission or failure to act on behalf of a child" (p. 414). There are three categories of abuse a therapeutic recreation specialist needs to be aware of: physical abuse, sexual abuse, and emotional abuse. The act of having to watch a parent be abused by the other parent may also be classified as abuse. Most symptoms of abused or neglected children are non-specific, but the children may be classified as developmentally delayed due to emotional problems, passive, overly aggressive, or other problems. Therapeutic recreation specialists can help these children gain coping skills and self-awareness. Also the children can gain the ability to express their emotions appropriately.

Antisocial behaviors, such as bullying, are also behavioral impairments. Persons who display "bullying" behavior may need help with self-esteem, and the family may need professional assistance. Delinquency and criminal behavior can also fall under this subcategory. These individuals usually display patterns of behavior that are not socially acceptable. Most of these individuals can be found in schools or institutions and prisons (American Psychiatric Association, 2000; Baglin, Lewis, & Williams, 2004; Carter, van Andel, & Robb, 2003; Mobily & MacNeil, 2002).

Addictions is the last competency in *Diagnostic Groupings and Populations Served.*

Many addictions start out as harmless pastimes, such as gambling or internet use. Perhaps the most well known addiction is drug abuse.

Polysubstance and alcohol dependence are both included within this subtopic. According to the American Psychiatric Association (2000), 11 classes of substances make up this category: "alcohol; amphetamines; caffeine; cannabis; cocaine; hallucinogens; inhalants; nicotine; opioids; phencyclidine; and sedatives, hypnotics or anxiolytics" (p. 191). Prescribed and over-the-counter medications can also be addictive. Substance abuse occurs when an individual repeatedly uses a substance to the point that it causes serious problems in life, whether it be problems on the job, in role obligations, legal problems, health, etc. Chemical dependency involves developing a reliance on one or a combination of drugs. Addiction is continued use of a drug to the point of a compulsion. At some point, addiction can become so serious that getting and using the drug is the focus of the person's life. It is a good idea to have an understanding of the different types of drugs found in each category, the symptoms of drug abuse, and the effects of leisure education on the recovery of persons who are dependent on polysubstances and alcohol. It is also a good idea to have an understanding of the treatment protocol for persons who are addicted to polysubstances and/or alcohol. The family system is impacted greatly by persons who are addicted to polysubstances and/or alcohol. The entry-level professional is expected to have an understanding of the impact on the family, co-dependent behavior, and potential family treatment.

People are not just addicted to drugs and alcohol. People can be addicted to gambling, exercise, work, etc. Gambling is becoming a greater concern as casinos become prevalent across the nation. There are people who cannot make it through the day unless they have exercised and have determined how many miles they must run before going to bed. They will ignore their family, work and other leisure activities until they have gotten the necessary miles in. There are also people who are addicted to work. They do not go anywhere without taking work along on vacation and making sure they are connected to the office through the internet. In summary, according to Kraus & Shank (1992), "…addiction represents a powerful kind of attraction, for what may initially appear to be a harmless kind of pleasure or personal release, but ultimately totally controls the individual and leads to shattering life consequences" (p. 319). All persons who are addicted could use goal-oriented treatment, leisure education, and an understanding of their behavior and how it affects others, especially the family (American Psychiatric Association, 2000; Carter, van Andel, & Robb, 2003; Faulkner, 1991; Kraus & Shank, 1992; Mobily & MacNeil, 2002; O'Dea-Evans, 1990).

Usually the information covered in this Knowledge Area is covered in a therapeutic recreation introductory class or a recreation for special population course. However, some colleges and universities offer special courses in therapeutic recreation that cover disabilities only.

References Related to Diagnostic Groups and Populations Served

American Psychiatric Association. (2000). *Diagnostic and statistical manual of mental disorders* (4th ed.). Washington, D.C.: Author.

Baglin, C. A., Lewis, M. E. B., & Williams B. (2004). *Recreation and leisure for persons with emotional problems and challenging behaviors.* Champaign, IL: Sagamore Publishing.

Bender, M., & Baglin, C. A., (2004). *Implementing recreation and leisure opportunities for infants and toddlers with disabilities.* Champaign, IL: Sagamore Publishing.

Buettner L., & Fitzsimmons, S. (2003). *Dementia practice guideline for recreational therapy: Treatment of disturbing behaviors.* Alexandria, VA: American Therapeutic Recreation Association.

Carter, M. J., & LeConney, S. P. (2004). *Therapeutic recreation in the community: An inclusive approach* (2nd ed.). Champaign, IL: Sagamore Publishing.

Carter, M. J., van Andel, G. E., & Robb, G. M. (2003). *Therapeutic recreation: A practical approach* (3rd ed.). Prospect Heights, IL: Waveland Press.

Coyne, P., & Fullerton, A. (2004). *Supporting individuals with autism spectrum disorder in recreation.* Champaign, IL: Sagamore Publishing.

Hawkins, B. A., May, M. E., & Rogers, N. B. (1996). *Therapeutic activity intervention with the elderly: Foundations & practices.* State College, PA: Venture Publishing.

Kraus, R., & Shank, J. (1992). *Therapeutic recreation service: Principles and practices* (4th ed.). Dubuque, IA: Wm. C. Brown & Co.

McGuire, F. A., Boyd, R. K., & Tedrick, R. E. (2004). *Leisure and aging: Ulyssean living in later life* (3rd ed.). Champaign, IL: Sagamore Publishing.

Mobily, K. E., & MacNeil, R. D. (2002). *Therapeutic recreation and the nature of disabilities.* State College, PA: Venture Publishing.

O'Dea-Evans, P. (1990). *Leisure education for addicted persons.* Algonquin, IL: Peapod Productions.

Tamparo, D. D., & Lewis, M. A. (2000). *Diseases of the human body* (3rd ed.). Philadelphia, PA: F. A. Davis Company.

Wilhite, B. C., & Keller, M. J. (2000). *Therapeutic recreation: Cases and exercises.* State College, PA: Venture Publishing.

Websites Related to Diagnostic Groupings and Populations Served

There are many websites that present information on various impairments. The following are a few that may provide you with more information.

The ARC (formerly the Association for Retarded Citizens) **www.thearc.org**
American Association for Mental Retardation **www.aamr.org**
Autism Society **www.autism-society.org**
American Stroke Association **www.strokeassociation.org**
National Association of Neurological Disorders and Strokes **www.ninds.nih.gov/health_and_medical/disorders**
Institute for Brain Aging and Dementia **www.alz.uci.edu**
Dementia **www.dementia.com**
Epilepsy **www.epilepsy.com**
Muscular Dystrophy Association **www.mdausa.org**
United Cerebral Palsy **www.ucpa.org**
National Multiple Sclerosis Society **www.nmss.org**
Cardiac **www.heartassociation.org**
American Diabetes Association **www.diabetes.org**
American Cancer Association **www.cancer.org**
HIV/AIDS Resources **www.aids.org** **www.thebody.com**
National Federation for the Blind **www.nfb.org**
American Foundation for the Blind **www.afb.org**
American Council for the Blind **www.acb.org**
National Association for the Deaf **www.nad.org**
Alexander Graham Bell Association for the Deaf and Hard of Hearing **www.agbell.org**

U.S. Department of Health & Human Services Center for Substance Abuse Prevention **www.samhsa.gov**
Alcoholism **www.alcoholism.about.com**

Assessment

Assessment is an important knowledge area for the entry-level therapeutic recreation specialist. Approximately 15 percent or 13 questions will focus on client assessment. The questions will not only cover the process and procedures of assessment, but the different assessments currently being used in the field. You need to have an understanding of the domains to be assessed, what to assess in those domains, basic assessment procedures, and the process of determining an appropriate assessment.

Looking at the competencies listed under Assessment, it is easy to see that assessment procedures, i.e., observation, interviewing and functional skills testing, current TR or leisure assessments, and other inventories and questionnaires are the first knowledge items in this category. The tools of observation, interviewing, and functional skills testing are three of the most important tools an entry-level therapist can have.

When observing a patient, the therapeutic recreation specialist must be able to sift through all the information the client may give and determine what is most important, dependent, of course, on the needs of the patient and the type of program (i.e., functional intervention, leisure education, etc.) that the therapeutic recreation department offers. Systematic observation is the most frequently used type of observation in the field today. It standardizes the procedures used, including identifying the targeted behavior, developing specific recording techniques for the observation of the targeted behavior and scoring and interpreting the observation. There are different types of recording methods/techniques used in therapeutic recreation including: checklists, rating scales, anecdotal records along with frequency or tally methods, and duration, interval and instantaneous time sampling techniques (Burlingame & Blaschko, 2002; Stumbo, 2002; Stumbo & Peterson, 2004).

The entry-level therapeutic recreation specialist needs to understand and use interview skills, keeping in mind the purpose of assessment interviews, which is to gather information about a client. There are two approaches to interviewing, directive and non-directive. Most therapeutic recreation specialists use the directive approach, which involves a series of questions targeted for a specific end result. Different types of questions can be asked in the interview, ranging from closed-ended questions (i.e., "What is your favorite leisure activity?") to open-ended questions (i.e., "Tell me what you like to do for fun."). A rule of thumb for interview questions is that they should directly relate to the purpose of the interview/assessment. Every interview should have an opening, a body of the interview, and a closing. All therapeutic recreation departments should have developed an interview protocol to use in assessment to ensure everyone is collecting the necessary information in the same way (Austin, 2004; Burlingame & Blaschko, 2002; Stumbo, 2002; Stumbo & Peterson, 2004).

For functional skills testing, in addition to needing both observation and interview skills, the therapeutic recreation specialist needs to be able to use mechanical measurement tools (i.e., stop-watches, measuring tapes or other objects) that will provide standardized information (Burlingame & Blaschko, 2002). Functional skills will be addressed further in

the social, physical, cognitive, and emotional domains of assessment.

Although many TR departments use their own agency-specific assessment, there are a variety of published therapeutic recreation/leisure assessments ranging from functional to leisure-based. It is important that as a therapeutic recreation specialist you are familiar with a variety of assessment instruments. These assessments range from functional assessments (e.g., the Ohio Scales of Leisure Functioning, the Comprehensive Evaluation in Recreation Therapy (CERT), and the Functional Assessment of Characteristics for Therapeutic Recreation (FACTR)) to leisure assessments and checklists (e.g., Leisure Diagnostic Battery (LDB), the Leisure Competence Measure (LCM), and the Leisurescope Plus). It is recommended that the entry-level professional review the assessments provided in several therapeutic recreation textbooks.

There are also other inventories and questionnaires an entry-level therapeutic recreation specialist needs to be aware of because they may contribute to the assessment of the patient, dependent on the agency where the therapeutic recreation specialist is working, or the therapeutic recreation specialist may be expected to understand the meaning of the results of these assessments for use in programming. These assessments include the Functional Independence Measure (FIM), the American Spinal Injury Association Scale (ASIA), the Rancho Los Amigos Scale and the Glasgow Coma Scale and the Children's Coma Scale, which are used primarily in rehabilitation units and hospitals. In order to receive Medicare reimbursement, inpatient physical rehabilitation hospitals and units are required to use the Inpatient Rehabilitation Facility-Patient Assessment Instrument (IRF-PAI). The

FIM is imbedded within the IRF-PAI. In many long-term care facilities, professionals may use the Global Deterioration Scale (GDS), the Mini-Mental State Examination, and for Medicare reimbursement they must use the Minimum Data Set for Resident Assessment and Care Screening (MDS). In psychiatric settings, the therapists need to understand the Multiaxial Assessment System, specifically the Global Assessment of Functioning (GAF) (Burlingame & Blaschko, 2002; Shank & Coyle, 2002; Stumbo, 2002; Wilhite & Keller, 2000).

Assessment processes, referring to sources of assessment data, selection of the assessment, implementation of the assessment, and interpretation of the assessment data, are an important part of assessment. They make up the second major subtopic of knowledge areas in assessment.

Sometimes it is not possible for the patient to provide all the necessary information for a complete assessment. So, it is important that as an entry-level professional you know to use *other sources of assessment information* such as medical records, educational records, interviews with family and friends, and other members of the treatment team (Austin, 2004; Burlingame & Blaschko, 2002; Carter & LeConey, 2004; Shank & Coyle, 2002; Stumbo, 2002; Stumbo & Peterson, 2004).

In order to *select the most appropriate assessment tool,* you need to have an understanding of reliability, validity, usability, and practicability. According to Peterson and Stumbo (2000), "reliability refers to the estimate of the consistency of measurement" (p. 210). When implementing the assessment, it is important that you completely understand the assessment tool and are able to administer it with ease, following the directions that were given to ensure test reliability or consistency. Validity, on the other hand, refers to "the extent to which the assessment meets its

intended purpose" (Stumbo, 2002, p. 32). So, does the assessment measure what is necessary to place the patient in the appropriate program and has it been tested on the population in the agency for which it is intended? Usability and practicability involve whether the assessment is "doable" as far as time constraints, ease of use, cost, availability, and staff knowledge and ability (Burlingame & Blaschko, 2002; Peterson & Stumbo, 2000; Stumbo, 2002; Sylvester, Voelkl, & Ellis, 2001).

When *implementing the assessment,* it is important that you completely understand the assessment tool and are able to administer it with ease following the directions that were given to ensure test reliability. The therapeutic recreation specialist needs to easily use strategies of interviews, observations, self-administered questionnaires, and record reviews depending on the information desired. According to Stumbo (2002), there is a seven-step process for the assessment implementation process, including: 1) reviewing the assessment protocol, 2) preparing for assessment, 3) administering assessment to the patient, 4) analyzing or scoring the assessment results, 5) interpreting results for placement into programs, 6) documenting results of assessment, and 7) reassessing the patient as necessary/monitoring progress (p. 118).

After administering the assessment, it is important that you *interpret the assessment* correctly. If you have used a published assessment instrument, it is imperative that you interpret the assessment as the manual recommends. Scores need to be interpreted through norm-referenced or criterion-referenced means if they are published assessments.

The last topic in assessment relates to behavioral domains. In therapeutic recreation, we are concerned with the functioning level of the entire person, not just the dysfunctional part; so, we assess functional abilities in the following domains: sensory, cognitive, social, physical, and emotional. We also assess a client's/patient's leisure—knowledge, interests, and skills—and gather a variety of background information for each client.

The *sensory domain* looks at a patient's ability to see and hear. Can he/she see to read? Is it functional sight, or is the patient essentially blind? Can the person hear? How much can he or she hear? Is it better to sit to one side of the patient when working with him or her because his or her hearing is better on one side? Also, how is the person in relationship to tactile abilities? Are they tactile defensive?

When looking at clients'/patients' *cognitive domain* it is important to look at his/her functional abilities. Thus, in general, a therapeutic recreation specialist is concerned with a patient's memory, both long and short term, his/her ability to solve problems, and his/her attention span. We are also concerned with our patient's orientation, in other words, is he oriented to person, place, and time? Another big concern is safety awareness. Is the patient aware of danger and can he take care of himself in public? All of these are examples of functional skills that can be assessed in the cognitive domain.

The *social domain* is a unique assessment. Within this domain the therapeutic recreation specialist is concerned with whether patients have good communication/interactive skills. Can they initiate a conversation, maintain a conversation, and respond appropriately to questions? Likewise, are they able to maintain friendships, and can they develop a support network? All of these are examples of functional skills that can be assessed in the social domain.

In the *physical domain,* the behaviors are more explicit. Therapeutic recreation specialists assess a person's fitness, his/her gross motor and fine motor skills. They assess a

patient's eye–hand coordination and other functional skills.

The *emotional domain* may be a little more difficult to assess. When assessing emotional skills, a therapeutic recreation specialist wants to know what the patient's attitude is toward self. How does he or she express emotions? Can he or she express anger appropriately? These are considered functional skills in the emotional domain.

It is imperative that a therapeutic recreation specialist assess a patient's *leisure functioning.* What leisure barriers does the person have? What are his leisure interests? What are her leisure attitudes? What leisure skills does the person have, and is she well rounded? What does the person know about leisure and is he able to get his leisure needs met? These are some of the areas to be assessed in the leisure domain.

The last area presented here is not actually a domain but rather *background information* that the therapeutic recreation specialist needs to have in order to effectively understand/use some of the information. In other words, one needs some basic demographics about patients (e.g., age, educational level, diagnosis, family, etc.). It is also important to gain an understanding of the patient's past medical history. Multicultural considerations such as the patient's cultural belief system are also important to keep in mind when assessing a patient. The therapeutic recreation specialist needs to "develop cultural self-awareness, use interpreters/translators and involve the family network" (Sylvester, Voelkl, & Ellis, 2001, pp. 138-139) to fully understand the implications of the assessment (Carter & LeConey, 2004).

Information on assessment is found throughout therapeutic recreation curriculum. It may be found in a separate course, such as Assessment and Evaluation in Therapeutic Recreation. It may be found within foundation courses or programming courses. It is a necessity in all therapeutic recreation curriculum as it provides the therapeutic recreation specialist with the necessary information to provide the required interventions.

References Related to Assessment

Austin, D. R. (2004). *Therapeutic recreation: Processes and techniques* (5th ed.). Champaign, IL: Sagamore Publishing.

Burlingame, J. & Blaschko, T. M. (2002). *Assessment tools for recreational therapy* (3rd ed.). Ravensdale, WA: Idyll Arbor.

Carter, M. J., & LeConey, S. P. (2004). *Therapeutic recreation in the community: An inclusive approach* (2nd ed.). Champaign, IL: Sagamore Publishing.

Shank, J., & Coyle, C. (2002). *Therapeutic recreation in health promotion and rehabilitation.* State College, PA: Venture Publishing.

Stumbo, N. J. (2002). *Client assessment in therapeutic recreation services.* State College, PA: Venture Publishing.

Stumbo, N. J., & Peterson, C. A. (2004). *Therapeutic recreation program design: Principles and procedures* (4th ed.). San Francisco: Benjamin Cummings.

Sylvester, C., Voelkl, J. E., & Ellis, G. D. (2001). *Therapeutic recreation programming: Theory and practice.* State College, PA: Venture Publishing.

Wilhite, B. C., & Keller, M. J. (2000). *Therapeutic recreation: Cases and exercises* (2nd ed.). State College, PA: Venture Publishing.

Planning the Intervention

The fourth knowledge area is *Planning the Intervention*, which will contribute 15 percent or 14 questions to the national exam. There are 16 competencies in this area and it is an important area in therapeutic recreation. It is within this Knowledge Area that one finds standards of practice, goals and objectives, codes of ethics, activity analysis, leisure education, and a variety of other competencies.

Understanding the impact the impairment has on the individual and the family is the first competency within Planning the Intervention. Any impairment that occurs will have an impact on the individual's life and the lives of the people who love and care for that individual. A person cannot assume that if a disability is physical in nature, that only that area of the individual's life will be impacted. Most likely the disability will present the person with secondary impairments, such as a changing social life that can then create other emotional problems. It may also create difficulties in his or her role in the family and in the world of work. Because most people who have a disability also have a family, this disability, whether it be a congenital disability or from trauma or disease, will impact other people. When working with a person with a disability, the therapeutic recreation professional needs to keep in mind that the entire family may need assistance in coping and then learning to accept and manage all the new information and skills now necessary (Kraus & Shank, 1992).

A therapeutic recreation specialist must also have an understanding of the concepts of *normalization, inclusion, and least restrictive environment* and what they mean in terms of programming. When thinking of "normalization" one must keep in the mind that persons with disabilities have the same needs and desires as persons who do not have disabilities. Thus, in regard to recreation and leisure service, normalization would imply that persons with disabilities should have the same opportunities that anyone without a disability in the community has. Their lives should be as typical as possible: going to school or work, participating in recreation activities, etc., with the same life cycle of activities, expectations and opportunities (i.e., attending dances, getting married, etc.).

Inclusion refers to a process that "enables an individual to be part of his environment by making choices, being supported in what he does on a daily basis, having friends, and being valued" (Bullock & Mahon, 2001, p. 58). Recreation has accepted the idea and now tries to present community activities as inclusive recreation. According to Dattilo (2002), when we embrace inclusion we "recognize we are one, yet we are different, create chances for others to experience freedom to participate, value each person and value diversity, and support participation" (p. 26). Community recreation programs are hiring therapeutic recreation specialists to enable persons with disabilities to participate in any community recreation program. The therapeutic recreation specialist may provide assistance through recommendations of leadership needs, activity or equipment adaptation or by providing support to assist everyone in accepting the person with a disability in the program. The therapeutic recreation specialist may not be needed after making the necessary program, equipment, or leadership adjustments.

The term "least restrictive environment" is an educational term that was first used in the Education of All Handicapped Children Act of 1975 (PL 94-142) and is part of the Individuals with Disabilities Education Act (IDEA). It refers to placing a child in a program where he can have the greatest success. Not all children are alike and that is also true of children with disabilities. Previously recreation programs may have created "segregated programming" for children with disabilities thinking this would serve those persons best; however, it is now recognized that children need a program that best fits their needs. For some individuals it may be segregated programming at first and then, when appropriate skills have been developed, move into inclusive programming. For other individuals it may always be segregated programming and, for others inclusive programming may be appropriate (Bullock & Mahon, 2001; Carter & LeConey, 2004; Dattilo, 2002; Kraus & Shank, 1992).

Architectural barriers and accessibility of programs are programming issues. According to Gorham and Brasile (1998) there are three components of accessibility ". . .architectural accessibility, program accessibility, and the skills required to access the resources now available to persons with disabilities" (p. 324). In 1965, the National Commission on Architectural Barriers was established. It recognized guidelines for architectural accessibility that were developed by the American National Standards Institute (ANSI). Currently, recreation facility planners must follow the standards issued by the American Transportation Barriers Compliance Board and those contained in the Uniform Federal Accessibility Standards and the Americans Disabilities Act Accessibility Guidelines (Dattilo, 2002). It is up to the therapeutic recreation specialist to be aware of the standards and to ensure that all recreation areas are as accessible as possible.

The National Center for Accessibility located in Bloomington, Indiana, works to ensure that there are appropriate accessibility guidelines established for recreation areas and facilities.

According to Gorham and Brasile (1998), program accessibility "focuses on the design and implementation of specific activities and other events" (p. 331). How does one provide accessible programming? Just because a facility is accessible does not mean the program is. In addition to the elimination of architectural barriers, the therapeutic recreation specialist must make sure there is appropriate transportation or access to the program, that activities have a range of skill levels and appropriate adaptations, that the fee for the program does not keep people with a limited income from participating and, that the program has been advertised to all people, including people who are deaf and may need interpreters or people who are blind and may need guides (Bullock & Mahon, 2001; Dattilo, 2002; Gorham & Brasile, 1998; Smith, Austin, & Kennedy, 2001).

The next competency in programming issues relates to *societal attitudes and stereotyping.* As an entry-level professional, you need to understand society's attitudes and what you can do to help educate and thus eliminate some of these attitudes. What is an attitude? "An attitude is a disposition to respond favorably or unfavorably to an object, person, institution or event" (Ajzen, 1988, p. 4). Attitudes can impact behavior. For years, society focused on individuals' differences, thus causing people to be unaware of how alike we are. This focus on differences caused fear and negative attitudes. Educating people about how alike we are is one purpose of therapeutic recreation specialists, thus helping to eliminate negative attitudes. Stereotyp-ing people with disabilities is also a programming issue. When we stereotype, we place everyone

into a group and fail to treat them as individuals. When we program, we must keep in mind individual needs and differences (Bedini, 1998; Bullock & Mahon, 2001; Dattilo, 2002; Smith, Austin, & Kennedy, 2001).

Perhaps the greatest impact on programming for people with disabilities has come from the government in the form of *legislation,* which is another competency in Planning the Intervention. There are a variety of pieces of legislation that have impacted people with disabilities in the United States and made access to recreation and therapeutic recreation services mandatory. Presented below are only the "highlights" of the laws that impact therapeutic recreation services.

- PL 93-112—The Rehabilitation Act of 1973
  - Title II trained recreation workers to work with people with disabilities and provided research money for recreation projects.
  - Section 304 made money available for demonstrating how to make recreation activities accessible.
  - Section 502 established the Architectural and Transportation Barriers Compliance Board.
  - Section 504–Nondiscrimination under Federal Grants. This is considered to be landmark legislation for individuals with disabilities and laid the groundwork for the Americans with Disabilities Act. It essentially said that a person with a disability could not be discriminated against in any program supported with federal monies.
- PL95-602—The Rehabilitation Act of 1978
  - Section 311 provided grants for operating and where necessary, removing or constructing facilities to demonstrate methods of making recreational activities accessible.

- Section 316 provided money to pay for the initiation of new recreation programs to provide activities to assist individuals with mobility and socialization.
- PL 94-142—The Education of All Handicapped Children Act of 1975
  - Ensured children with disabilities a free and appropriate education.
  - Included recreation as a "related service" defining it as including:
    - assessment of recreation and leisure functioning,
    - leisure education,
    - therapeutic recreation, and
    - recreation in school and community agencies.
  - Required parents and teachers to write an Individualized Education Plan for all children with disabilities.
- PL 101-476—Individuals with Disabilities Education Act of 1990 (amendments to The Education of All Handicapped Children Act—changing the name)
  - Required more fully the inclusion of children with autism and traumatic brain injury.
  - Includes transition and assistive technology services.
- PL 105-117—Individuals with Disabilities Education Act of 1997 (reauthorization with amendments)
  - Behavioral plans must be developed.
  - Transition services need to be included beginning at age 14.
- PL 101-336—The Americans with Disabilities Act of 1990
  - Defines person with a disability as an individual who
    - has a physical or mental impairment that substantially limits one or more major life activities,
    - has a record of such an impairment, and

—is regarded as having such an impairment.
  - Disability has to result in a substantial limitation of one or more major life activities.
  - Four Primary Titles under the ADA
    Title I. Employment
    Title IIA. Government Services
    Title IIB. Public Transit
    Title III. Public Accommodation
    Title IV. Telecommunications
- New Freedom Initiative of 2000
  - Increasing access to assistive and universally designed technologies.
  - Expanding educational opportunities for Americans with disabilities.
  - Promoting full access to community life.

You need to understand the provisions of these important pieces of legislation because they have had, and will continue to have, an impact on the lives of persons with disabilities and therapeutic recreation/recreation services (Bullock & Mahon, 2001; Carter, van Andel, & Robb, 2003; Dattilo, 2002; Kraus & Shank, 1992; Lawson, Coyle, & Ashton-Shaeffer, 2001).

Understanding and knowing the *Standards of Practice for the Therapeutic Recreation Profession* is very important for the entry-level professional, for these standards are what must guide their practice. As an entry-level professional, you need to understand that there are two different written documents labeled *Standards of Practice for the Therapeutic Recreation Profession,* one was developed by the National Therapeutic Recreation Society (NTRS) and the other was developed by the American Therapeutic Recreation Association (ATRA). It is likely that if there is a test question from one publication, there will be a question from the other. The organization and presentation of the two documents are quite different, although the content, of course, is quite similar as both documents define the scope of service of the therapeutic recreation profession. It is recommended that you are familiar with both documents and know how they are alike and different. Both organizations have written documents that assist the practitioner in understanding and utilizing their standards of practice (ATRA, 1991, 2001; NTRS, 1994, 2003). (Now on web site).

Understanding and following a *Code of Ethics of the Therapeutic Recreation Profession* is an important aspect of programming since it guides professional behavior. A code of ethics is essentially a standard of behavior that is expected of all professionals. The field of therapeutic recreation has two codes of ethics for the profession; both NTRS (1990) and ATRA (2001) have developed codes of ethics and interpretative guidelines. These codes of ethics are self-regulatory but are developed to govern behavior. Copies of the Codes of Ethics of both professional organizations can be found on their web sites (ATRA, 1998; Jacobson, 2001; NTRS, 1994; Shank & Coyle, 2002; Spielman, 1998; Sylvester, Voelkl, & Ellis, 2001).

The next competency is related to the *nature and diversity of recreation and leisure activities*. Understanding the range of activities from outdoor to board and table games to spectator sports and the breadth of activities within those categories gives a professional a greater depth of knowledge thus able to provide a more diverse and, perhaps, needed program for clients/patients (Wilhite & Keller, 2000).

You need to be able to determine which activity would be the most appropriate for a specific program and why one program would be more appropriate for a specific client population than another. An understanding of the

purpose and use of *activity analysis* in programming is a necessity. Activity analysis helps the therapeutic recreation specialist examine its physical, social, emotional, and cognitive requirements in order to determine the skills, equipment, and materials necessary to successfully participate in the activity. Thus, activity analysis enables a therapeutic recreation specialist to determine if an activity is appropriate for the patient at the patient's current skill level or if the activity will assist the patient in reaching his/her goals. In other words, which activity will provide the greatest benefit for the patient? After completing an activity analysis, the activity can be modified if needed, to assist the client/patient in meeting specific goals. Several activity analysis forms have been developed and can be found in the textbooks listed at the end of this section (Austin, 2004; Stumbo & Peterson, 2004; Sylvester, Voelkl, & Ellis, 2001; Wilhite & Keller, 2000).

When planning a program, the therapeutic recreation specialist must understand the impact of *relevant guidelines and standards*. This means that you need to be aware of federal and state regulatory agencies, accrediting bodies, and payment systems that may impact the program. As the therapeutic recreation specialist is designing the program, it is important to be aware that legislation such as the ADA has an influence on community recreation programming, since no person can be refused due to a disability. Also, facilities that receive Medicare funding must follow the regulations established by the Centers for Medicare and Medicaid Services (CMS) (formerly the Health Care Financing Administration). The Joint Commission on Accreditation of Healthcare Organizations (JCAHO) and the Rehabilitation Accreditation Commission (CARF) are agencies that provide accreditation for hospitals and agencies that provides health care services. JCAHO sets standards for the following groups of healthcare agencies that might offer therapeutic recreation services: ambulatory care, assisted living, behavioral health care, health care networks, managed behavioral health care, preferred provider organizations, home care, hospitals, and long-term care. In order to become accredited by JCAHO, the hospital or healthcare agency must meet established standards. These standards have a strong influence on programming. CARF also establishes standards for hospitals and a variety of healthcare organizations that might offer therapeutic recreation services including: adult day services, assisted living standards, behavioral health, blind rehabilitation, employment and community services, and medical rehabilitation. The standards developed by CARF also address programming issues (Stumbo & Peterson, 2004; Sylvester, Voelkl, & Ellis, 2001).

Leisure education assists people in regaining a fulfilling leisure lifestyle and may help them understand the importance of leisure in their life, or gain a new leisure skill. Leisure education is an important part of a program because it is an area that is often forgotten when working with patients in a hospital or heath care agency, and is sorely needed when the patient returns home. In the hospital, much of the time is programmed, but at home, it is not. Many people will return home and be unable to return to work. Leisure education can help patients/clients understand the importance of using leisure wisely, developing a healthy leisure lifestyle, expanding their knowledge of leisure activities, and developing new skills. Patients may have participated in many leisure activities previously, but for one reason or another may not be participating in them now. Leisure education can help them learn how to adapt activities or determine any specialized equipment needed to participate. Leisure education can also help with learning about and utilizing leisure resources. These resources can range from personal resources to community resources or even activity opportunities (Bullock & Mahon, 2001; Dattilo, 1999; Shank & Coyle, 2002; Stumbo & Peterson, 2004).

The *selection of programs, activities, and interventions to achieve the assessed needs of the person* served is another important competency. According to Shank and Coyle (2001), "you will need an understanding of three things: clients, activity-based interventions, and yourself" (p. 157). Based on the assessment of each client and from the treatment team, a list of client needs can be developed. You need to have knowledge of a wide variety of activities and interventions. Using activity analysis, you should be able to determine the appropriate activity for a client/patient and the intervention strategy to be used. When determining programs, activities and interventions, it is useful to review the diagnostic protocol that has been developed for each diagnosis and the program protocol that has been developed for each program. Determining program, activities, and interventions will also depend on the agency philosophy, type of program, space available, resources available, and length of stay and frequency of involvement in the therapeutic recreation program. Clinical practice guidelines are now under development for many diagnostic groups, which will help practice become more standardized. As of mid 2004 only *Dementia Practice Guidelines* (Buettner & Fitzsimmons, 2003) have been published and widely accepted (Carter, van Andel, & Robb, 2003; Shank & Coyle, 2001; Stumbo & Peterson, 2004; Sylvester, Voelkl, & Ellis, 2001; Wilhite & Keller, 2000).

When designing the program it is also important to determine any *assistive techniques or adaptive technology needed* by the client in order to become more independent. After understanding the needs of the patient and completing an activity analysis, the therapeutic recreation specialist should be able to make accurate activity modifications and determine necessary assistive techniques and equipment. These could range from simple card holders to adapted fishing poles to specialized wheelchairs to computer based devices (Broach, Dattilo, & Deavours, 2000; Bullock & Mahon, 2001; Dattilo, 2002; Paciorek & Jones, 2001; Williams, 2004).

One of the most important skills a therapeutic recreation specialist needs to have is to be able to write *measurable goals and behavioral objectives.* Based on the client's strengths and weaknesses as determined by the assessment, measurable goals and behavioral objectives are written. Goals flow directly from the needs list and are statements that reflect what the client is going to be able to do at the completion of that aspect of his/her treatment plan. For example, an outcome goal might be: To increase social interaction skills.

Based on the goal statement, behavioral objectives will be written. These behavioral objectives are indicators that a goal has been achieved. Objectives (sometimes referred to as outcome measures) must have three components: 1) conditions that state when or where the outcome behavior should occur, 2) an action verb that describes the expected behavior, and 3) criteria that describes how well the client must perform the behavior. Thus, based on the above stated goal, an appropriate outcome measure or objective might be: When asked a question by staff the client will respond politely within 30 seconds. The conditions are "when asked a question by staff", the action verb is "will respond," and the criteria

are "politely within 30 seconds." Writing good behavioral objectives takes practice. You may find that during your internship, shortcuts were taken by the therapeutic recreation staff. Please understand that those "short cuts" are not universally acceptable (Carter, van Andel, & Robb, 2003; Melcher, 1999; Shank & Coyle, 2002; Stumbo & Peterson, 2004; Sylvester, Voelkl, & Ellis, 2001).

The next competency expects the entry-level professional to have an *understanding of the roles and functions of other health and human service professionals and of interdisciplinary approaches.* The therapeutic recreation specialist is expected to understand the roles of treatment team members, such as psychiatric social workers or psychiatrists and their roles in the rehabilitation process. Most therapeutic recreation specialists will co-treat with other professionals on the treatment team and need to understand what each discipline can provide in the treatment process. For example, the physical therapist and the therapeutic recreation specialist may co-treat on a community re-integration program with the physical therapist working on car transfers or walking endurance, while the therapeutic recreation specialist is working on decision making, community resources, or money management skills.

Use of quality/performance improvement guidelines in program planning and implementation is the last competency in this Knowledge Area. Quality or performance improvement refers to the efforts of health care personnel to constantly be offering improved patient care. These are usually formal administrative procedures that must be considered in the development of programs. For example, if one of the standards established by the agency for quality/performance improvement is that all newly admitted patients will be assessed within the first 48 hours, then that also needs to be stated within the therapeutic recreation department's policies and procedures and built into the overall program. Essentially quality/performance improvement is an evaluative activity, and as such, the information received should be used to improve program performance (McCormick, 2003; Stumbo & Peterson, 2004). Further information on quality/performance improvement is found in other Knowledge Areas.

Information on this Knowledge Area can be found in introductory classes and upper division classes that deal directly with program planning in therapeutic recreation. It is recommended that you practice writing treatment plans and that you also practice developing therapeutic recreation programs in all program areas: functional intervention, leisure education, community reintegration, and recreation. Your internship should also have prepared you for this Knowledge Area.

References Related to Planning the Intervention

Ajzen, I. (1988). *Attitudes, personality and behavior.* Chicago, IL: The Doresey Press.

American Therapeutic Recreation Association. (2001). *Standards for the practice of therapeutic recreation and self-assessment guide.* Alexandria, VA: Author.

American Therapeutic Recreation Association. (1998). *Finding the path: Ethics in action.* Hattiesburg, MS: Author.

American Therapeutic Recreation Association. (1998). *Code of ethics.* Alexandria, VA: Author.

American Therapeutic Recreation Association. (1991). *Standards for the practice of therapeutic recreation.* Alexandria, VA: Author.

Austin, D. R. (2004). *Therapeutic recreation: Processes and techniques* (5th ed.). Champaign, IL: Sagamore Publishing.

Bedini, L. (1998). Attitudes toward disability. In F. Brasile, T. K. Skalko, & J. Burlingame, (Eds.), *Perspectives in recreational therapy: Issues of a dynamic profession* (pp. 287-309). Ravensdale, WA: Idyll Arbor.

Broach, E., Dattilo, J., & Deavours, M. (2000). Assistive technology. In J. Dattilo (Ed.), *Facilitation techniques in therapeutic recreation* (pp. 99-132). State College, PA: Venture Publishing.

Buettner, L., & Fitzsimmons, S. (2003). *Dementia practice guideline for recreational therapy: Treatment of disturbing behaviors.* Alexandria, VA: American Therapeutic Recreation Association.

Bullock, C. C., & Mahon, M. J. (2001). *Introduction to recreation services for people with disabilities: A person-centered approach* (2nd ed.). Champaign, IL: Sagamore Publishing.

Carter, M. J., & LeConey, S. P. (2004). *Therapeutic recreation in the community: An inclusive approach* (2nd ed.). Champaign, IL: Sagamore Publishing.

Carter, M. J., van Andel, G. E., & Robb, G. M. (2003). *Therapeutic recreation: A practical approach* (3rd ed.). Prospect Heights, IL: Waveland Press.

Dattilo, J. (2002). *Inclusive leisure services: Responding to the rights of people with disabilities* (2nd ed.). State College, PA: Venture Publishing.

Dattilo, J. (1999). *Leisure education program planning: A systematic approach* (2nd ed.). State College, PA: Venture Publishing.

Gorham, P., & Brasile, F. (1998). Accessibility: A bridge to a more inclusive community. In F. Brasile, T. K. Skalko, & J. Burlingame

(Eds.), *Perspectives in recreational therapy: Issues of a dynamic profession* (pp. 323-342). Ravensdale, WA: Idyll Arbor, Inc.

Jacobson, J. M., & James, A. (2001). Ethics: Doing right. In N. J. Stumbo (Ed.), *Professional issues in therapeutic recreation: On competence and outcomes* (pp. 237-248). Champaign, IL: Sagamore Publishing.

Kraus, R., & Shank, J. (1992). *Therapeutic recreation service: Principles and practices.* Dubuque, IA: Wm. C. Brown.

Lawson, L. M., Coyle, C. P., & Ashton-Shaeffer, C. (2001). *Therapeutic recreation in special education: An IDEA for the future.* Alexandria, VA: American Therapeutic Recreation Association.

McCormick, B. P. (2003). Outcomes measurement as a tool for performance. In N. J. Stumbo (Ed.), *Client outcomes in therapeutic recreation services* (pp. 221-231). State College, PA: Venture Publishing.

Melcher, S. (1999). *Introduction to writing goals and objectives: A manual for recreation therapy students and entry-level professionals.* State College, PA: Venture Publishing.

National Therapeutic Recreation Society. (1994). *Code of ethics and interpretive guidelines.* Alexandria, VA: National Recreation and Park Association.

National Therapeutic Recreation Society. (1994). *Standards of practice for therapeutic recreation services.* Alexandria, VA: National Recreation and Park Association.

National Therapeutic Recreation Society. (2003). *Standards of practice for therapeutic recreation services.* Alexandria, VA: National Recreation and Park Association.

Paciorek, M. J., & Jones, J. A. (2001). *Disability sport and recreation resources* (3rd ed.). Traverse City, MI: Cooper Publishing.

Shank, J., & Coyle, C. (2002). *Therapeutic recreation in health promotion and rehabilitation.* State College, PA: Venture Publishing.

Smith, R., Austin, D., & Kennedy, D. (2001). *Inclusive and special recreation: Opportunities for persons with disabilities* (4th ed.). New York, NY: McGraw-Hill.

Spielman, M. B. (1998). Ethics: To do the right thing. In F. Brasile, T. K. Skalko, & J. Burlingame (Eds.), *Perspectives in recreational therapy: Issues of a dynamic profession* (pp. 63-80). Ravensdale, WA: Idyll Arbor, Inc.

Stumbo, N. J., & Peterson, C. A. (2004). *Therapeutic recreation program design: Principles and procedures* (4th ed.). San Francisco, CA: Pearson.

Sylvester, C., Voelkl, J. E., & Ellis, G. D. (2001). *Therapeutic recreation programming: Theory and practice.* State College, PA: Venture Publishing.

Wilhite, B. C., & Keller, M. J. (2001). *Therapeutic recreation: Cases and exercises* (2nd ed.). State College, PA: Venture Publishing.

Williams, B. (2004). *Assistive devices, adaptive strategies, and recreational activities for students with disabilities.* Champaign, IL: Sagamore Publishing.

Implementing the Individualized Intervention Plan

The fifth knowledge area is *Implementing the Individualized Intervention Plan* which will contribute 16 percent or 14 questions to the national exam. This section of the exam will be concerned with ensuring that the entry-level therapeutic recreation specialist has an understanding of group leadership principles, behavioral change principles, intervention techniques, and methods of educating and incorporating families and relevant others.

The first competency in this knowledge area is principles of group interaction and leadership. Being able to lead group intervention sessions is very important in the field of therapeutic recreation. Because many of our activities take place with groups, the entry-level therapist needs to have an understanding of groups. According to Shank and Coyle (2002), ". . .groups provide opportunities for interactions among clients and, recreation therapists use these interactions to facilitate therapeutic outcomes" (p. 211). Thus having an understanding of group structure, principles, and leadership is important. There are important structural elements in a group: size, format (closed or open groups), type of clients in a group, and duration of group (is it ongoing or does it cease functioning after so many meetings?). As a therapeutic recreation specialist, you're expected to be able to place clients in the most appropriate intervention group based on their needs and abilities. Group leaders need to be enthusiastic and be able to act as a link between individual group members and the group. Not only do therapeutic recreation therapists need to be able to lead specific activities, but they need to watch members for any potential problems, help with necessary activity adaptations, and engage the patient/client in discussions.

In structuring a group session, there are three important parts: the opening of the session, the body of the session, and the closing of the session. In the opening of the group session, the therapeutic recreation specialist helps the clients relax and get to know each other. Also the TRS lets the group members know what is going to occur during the session as far as the activity is concerned. The body is the focus of the group's session. Whether it is a game, an arts and crafts project, a leisure awareness activity, or an experiential activity, it is up to the TRS to be prepared with the activity ready to go. The TRS needs to keep in mind the outcomes of the activity and then facilitate the activity so the purpose and goals are attained. At the end of

the activity it is important to "process the activity." Processing involves talking with the clients about what they think, how they feel, and anything else that relates to the behavior displayed during the activity. Processing is a very important part of the session because it focuses on what just happened and can help the client generalize his/her behavior into other aspects of his/her life. In order to be able to process effectively, the TRS needs to be able to do the following: focus, redirect, block, link and summarize (Shank & Coyle, 2002). The TRS needs to be able to summarize and effectively bring closure to the session. It is the ability to utilize these leadership principles that will assist the therapeutic recreation specialist in providing a truly therapeutic session. No matter how many activities a person knows, if the activities are not led well, the client/patient will not benefit as much as possible (Austin, 2002; Austin, 2004; Shank & Coyle, 2002).

Theories of human behavior change were presented in the *Background* knowledge area. The competency, *principles of behavioral change,* will be presented here. Probably the most widely accepted method of behavioral change is the cognitive behavioral change process. There are essentially three components to this principle. The first component is "antecedents" which are the thoughts, perceptions, or beliefs that a person has about a topic or experience. The second component is "action" which is the actual behavior of the patient or client. The last component is "consequences," which refers to the actual response to the action. This response can reinforce the original thoughts, beliefs, or perceptions. The client will have specific beliefs or thoughts, and perceptions (antecedents) about something and behave in a way that displays those antecedents. The therapeutic recreation specialist will use a structured therapeutic recreation intervention that will have an impact on the outcome thus influencing the consequences (Dattilo & Murphy, 1987; Shank & Coyle, 2002).

A subtopic in this knowledge area is *Intervention Techniques.* There are many different interventions used in therapeutic recreation programs dependent upon the client population, needs of the client, agency philosophy, and program. The following techniques are not all inclusive, but are the ones from the NCTRC knowledge competency list. There are many more interventions used in therapeutic recreation.

Behavior management techniques include behavior modification and coping skills. Some people with whom therapeutic recreation specialists work have some behaviors that are problematic. Using behavior modification techniques to help patients/clients learn to manage their own behavior may be necessary. The following will be information on specific concepts of behavior modification. Positive reinforcement is the provision of a reinforcer that will cause the behavior to be repeated. A reinforcer is anything that causes a behavior to be repeated; it can be attention, food, etc. Punishment decreases the occurrence of a negative behavior. Modeling is the demonstration of desired behavior and combined with reinforcement, causes the patient/client to want to repeat the behavior. Time out is the removal of the child or individual from a reinforcer or stimulating event. It is used frequently with children who are having difficulty coping with an overstimulating environment. Token economies are used in some residential settings. Residents receive tokens for specified behaviors; at the end of a day or week those tokens can be redeemed for something of value to the individual (Austin, 2004; Dattilo & Wolfe, 2002; Dattilo & Murphy, 1987; Wilhite & Keller, 2000).

Learning to cope is also an important behavior management technique. All of us have stress, and learning to cope with stress is an area in which therapeutic recreation specialists are expected to be able to assist patients/clients. Coping should be a deliberate process and not an automatic adaptive behavior. The use of diversional activities can help people learn to cope with stressors. Some people have found that exercise can help an individual reduce tension and cope with stress. People can also learn to rely on social support systems to assist them in their coping skills (Shank & Coyle, 2002).

Stress seems to be a factor in everyone's life these days. Whether it's the stress of a job, the loss of a loved one, or the impact of a disability, the ability to teach clients to understand and *manage stress using relaxation techniques* is a function of the entry-level therapeutic recreation specialist. There are a variety of relaxation techniques that the therapeutic recreation specialist needs to understand and use. A few relaxation techniques include: deep-breathing exercises, progressive relaxation techniques, creative visualization, autogenic training, Tai Chi, and stretching (Austin, 2004; Carter, van Andel, & Robb, 2003; Shank & Coyle, 2002; Wilhite & Keller, 2000).

Teaching our clients *assertiveness skills* is an important intervention skill that a therapeutic recreation specialist needs to understand and be able to teach patients/clients. Assertiveness skills are useful in everyone's life, especially for individuals who have problems expressing their feelings or needs. Our patients need to learn the difference between passive, aggressive, and assertive behavior and learn to use assertive behavior in their interactions (Austin, 2004; Carter, van Andel, & Robb, 2003; Mascott, 2004; Shank & Coyle, 2002).

Remotivation is an intervention technique used with older adults in long-term care facilities. It encourages the individual to reestablish contact with the outside world by introducing topics of interest to the individual through group activities that encourage the use of verbal and cognitive skills, especially long-term memory. It usually occurs in a group setting and lasts from 30 minutes to an hour. There is a specific format used with remotivation and includes: 1) a climate of acceptance (introductions and welcome), 2) the bridge to reality (focusing attention on a specific topic by reading a poem, singing a song, etc.), 3) sharing the world we live in (inviting responses to specific questions based on the previously introduced topic), 4) appreciation of the work of the world (focuses on jobs and tasks familiar to them and related to the topic of the day), and 5) a climate of appreciation (summarization of the day's topic and discussion) (Austin, 2004; Carter, van Andel, & Robb, 2003; Hawkins, May, & Rogers, 1996; Shank & Coyle, 2002; Wilhite & Keller, 2000).

Reality orientation is also an intervention technique used with older adults who are confused, disoriented, and have memory loss. Reality orientation can occur all day through the use of a reality orientation board with basic facts like time, place, day of the week, date, next meal, next holiday, etc. It can also be run as a group with the therapeutic recreation specialists as the facilitators. In a group setting, the groups might review the facts on the board, use various activities to help diminish confusion review various aspects of activities of daily living (Austin, 2004; Carter, van Andel, & Robb, 2003; Hawkins, May, & Rogers, 1996; Shank & Coyle, 2002; Wilhite & Keller, 2000).

Cognitive retraining is used with people who have had a traumatic brain injury or CVA. It helps the person work on regaining some of the cognitive processes such as memory or sequencing that were injured or impaired. Various activities such as computer games and crafts that would rely on planning skills and decision-making skills are used in cognitive retraining groups. Cognitive retraining also teaches them to use a variety of compensatory strategies. If short-term memory is a problem, the client learns various memory techniques or how to effectively use assistive devices like using a personal data assistant (PDA) to keep track of important information (Austin, 2004; Carter, van Andel, & Robb, 2003; Shank & Coyle, 2002).

Counseling techniques are sometimes referred to in the literature as communication skills. Effective communication is important when working with patients/clients. One of the most important skills a therapeutic recreation specialist can have is the ability to listen; active listening lets the patient/client know you heard what was said. Listening skills are both verbal and non-verbal. Attending skills consist of the following non-verbal behaviors: eye contact, posture, and gestures; it also consists of various verbal behaviors, but primarily are the ones that keep the patient/client talking like "uh-huh" or "I see." There are also other verbal behaviors that let the patient/client know you are listening and encourage patients/clients to talk. They consist of: paraphrasing, clarifying, perception checking, probing, reflecting, interpreting, confronting, informing, self-disclosing, and summarizing. If you are not familiar with these counseling techniques, it is recommended that you review and practice them (Austin, 2004; Shank & Coyle, 2002; Sylvester, Voelkl, & Ellis, 2001).

Sensory stimulation is another intervention techniques used by therapeutic recreation specialists. It is used to bombard the senses with a variety of stimulants. Sensory stimulation may be used with older adults who are experiencing dementia or children with developmental or neurological deficits. The idea is to use sensory cues to relate to familiar life activities. Any one of the five senses is selected and the individual is expected to relate that sensual experience to the environment or to a memory. For example, a person is given a certain scent to smell and then asked to relate it to something in his past or present, like the scent of vanilla being related to baking (Austin, 2004; Hawkins, May, & Rogers, 1996; Shank & Coyle, 2002; Sylvester, Voelkl, & Ellis, 2001; Wilhite & Keller, 2000).

As stated earlier, it is not just the individual who is affected by the disability but the whole family. Thus, another competency is *methods for educating and incorporating families and relevant others.* It is the family who provides the support for the person with a disability and is also impacted by the disabling condition. Designing programs to include all members of the family is an important aspect of the job. A variety of materials from brochures to videos can be developed to explain the person's disabilities. Including these family members in your programming and if possible, some of your treatment programs, is important for everyone. Taking the patient/client on a community reentry outing with family members can help the family understand the needs of their family member. Including grandchildren in a game of cards may be motivating to the patient and also let the grandchild know that grandpa or grandma still wants to "play" with them (Austin, 2004; Shank & Coyle, 2002; Sylvester, Voelkl, & Ellis, 2001).

Validation intervention programs are used primarily with older adults experiencing dementia. It does not try to orient them to reality but to accept their feelings and assist the older adult in resolving unfinished business/conflicts experienced earlier in life. Its techniques are relatively simple, needing only the ability to accept people who are confused or disoriented for where they are right now and to use good listening and communication skills. It allows the older adult to express his feelings, acknowledge his life through reminiscence, and come to terms with his losses (Austin, 2004; Carter, van Andel, & Robb, 2003; Hawkins, May, & Rogers, 1996).

Values clarification techniques are used frequently in leisure education programs. Its requirements of choosing, cherishing, and acting on values have benefited persons who are chemically dependent, have psychiatric impairments—both adolescents and adults— or who have mental impairments. According to McKenney and Dattilo (2000), there are three value clarification strategies that are useful in leisure education: the individual clarifying response (help individuals think about what they just said or did), the group discussion (encourage reflection of the patient's ideas within a group setting), and value sheets (raise a value issue within a group) (Austin, 2004; Carter, van Andel, & Robb, 2003; McKenney & Dattilo, 2000).

Social skills training is used with persons who have psychiatric impairments, mental impairments, traumatic brain injuries, with many other populations. Many people within our society have problems with social interaction skills, understanding of the importance of friendship and how to make friends, the use of manners, etc. Since most recreation and leisure activities take place in a social situation, it is important for therapeutic recreation specialists to teach social skills to their patients/clients. Typically people who do social skills training use techniques such as modeling, role playing, social reinforcement, and homework used to practice learned skills in real-life situations (Austin, 2004; Carter, van Andel, & Robb, 2003; Shank, 2002).

This knowledge area, *Implementing the Individualized Intervention Plan,* expects the entry-level therapeutic recreation specialist to be able to actualize the treatment plan using a variety of leadership techniques and intervention strategies. Most of the knowledge and skills required in this knowledge area are taught in a techniques/interventions class. The list of intervention programs and activities listed here is by no means exhaustive. There are many more utilized in therapeutic recreation services. Your internship should have given you practice in implementing interventions and leading activities.

References Related to Implementing the Individualized Intervention Plan

Austin, D. R. (2004). *Therapeutic recreation: Processes and techniques* (5th ed.). Champaign, IL: Sagamore Publishing.

Austin, D. R. (2002). The therapeutic relationship. In D. R. Austin, J. Dattilo, & B. P. McCormick (Eds.), *Conceptual foundations for therapeutic recreation* (pp. 115-131). State College, PA: Venture Publishing.

Carter, M. J., van Andel, G. E., & Robb, G. M. (2003). *Therapeutic recreation: A practical approach* (3rd ed.). Prospect Heights, IL: Waveland Press.

Dattilo, J., & Murphy, W. D. (1987). *Behavior modification in therapeutic recreation.* State College, PA: Venture Publishing.

Dattilo, J. & Wolfe, B. (2002). Behavior modification in therapeutic recreation: Observing behaviors and applying consequences. In D. R. Austin, J. Dattilo, & B. P. McCormick (Eds.), *Conceptual foundations for therapeutic recreation* (pp. 31-47). State College, PA: Venture Publishing.

Hawkins, B. A., May, M. E., & Rogers, N. B. (1996). *Therapeutic activity intervention with the elderly: Foundations & practices.* State College, PA: Venture Publishing.

Mascott, C. (2004). *The therapeutic recreation stress management primer.* State College, PA: Venture Publishing.

McKenney, A., & Dattilo, J. (2000). Values clarification. In J. Dattilo, (Ed.), *Facilitation techniques in therapeutic recreation,* (pp. 477-495). State College, PA: Venture Publishing.

Shank J., & Coyle, C. (2002). *Therapeutic recreation in health promotion and rehabilitation.* State College, PA: Venture Publishing.

Sylvester, C., Voelkl, J. E., & Ellis, G. D. (2001). *Therapeutic recreation programming: Theory and practice.* State College, PA: Venture Publishing.

Wilhite, B. C., & Keller, M. J. (2000). *Therapeutic recreation: Cases and exercises* (2nd ed.). State College, PA: Venture Publishing.

Documentation and Evaluation

Documenting client progress and *evaluating* programs is an important aspect of a therapeutic recreation specialist's job. Although there are only five competencies in this knowledge area, it will provide 13 questions to the exam.

The first competency is *methods of documenting assessment, progress/functional status, discharge/transition plans of the person served.* After carefully assessing the patient, it is necessary to enter the assessment information into the medical chart or treatment plan. When documenting the assessment results, the TRS summarizes the assessment information. It is important to include information about the patient's strengths, weaknesses, the process used to collect the assessment information, and mutually agreed upon treatment goals and interventions. Each problem and strength needs to be written in measurable terminology; diagnostic labels (e.g., depressed) must not be used as a problem statement. The method of documentation used will determine the format of the assessment documentation. If it is Narrative, the assessment data can be written in narrative or paragraph format; if using Problem-Oriented Medical Records, it may be acceptable to list the information. Also placement of the assessment is dependent on whether the agency uses source-oriented records or problem-oriented records. If source oriented is used, the assessment information would be entered in the therapeutic recreation section of the chart; if problem oriented is used, assessment information will be entered in the assessment or data base section of the chart.

After entering assessment information, the TRS will enter progress notes dependent on the requirements of the agency. After working with a patient, the TRS must provide periodic updates on the patient's/client's progress toward meeting her goals. The frequency of providing updates on the patient's progress is determined by agency guidelines, accreditation standards, and regulatory agencies.

Different types of record-keeping systems are used for documentation, such as narrative charting, problem-oriented medical records (POMR), and charting by exception (CBE). Narrative charting is used frequently by community-based agencies, adult day-care facilities, and residential settings. Information must be about progress toward goals, but there is no uniform structure or format.

Problem-oriented medical records is a way to organize a chart. There are five components to this kind of medical record keeping: database (initial assessment results, client problem list, initial treatment plan, progress notes using SOAP, SOAPIE or SOAPIER, and a discharge summary). SOAP is a common form of charting progress notes and is primarily used in hospital settings. SOAP is an acronym that stands for **S**ubjective, **O**bjective, **A**nalysis and **P**lan. "Subjective" data is a direct quote from a patient; "Objective" is data that is gathered by observation of the patient's actions or behaviors; "Analysis" is the interpretation the TRS makes from the subjective and objective behavior; and, "Plan" is the plan that is recommended based on the previous information. SOAPIE adds "Intervention"—what specific intervention was used; and "Evaluation" is how the client responded to the intervention. SOAPIER adds "**R**evision" for changes made in the original treatment plan.

Charting by Exception (CBE) is used in agencies that have clearly detailed clinical pathways or long-term care facilities. When an agency has a clearly detailed clinical pathway that is being followed, the only time it is necessary to chart is when there is a variance or exception from the typical course of recovery. In a long-term care facility, as long as the person is not having any changes in functioning or health, there is no charting on the individual. These are only three examples of the types of charting used in agencies where therapeutic recreation specialists may work; there are many others. Computers also impact charting, and different software for electronic charting is being developed (Austin, 2004; Shank & Coyle, 2002; Stumbo & Peterson, 2004).

According to many people, discharge planning should begin the day the patient arrives on the unit. Discharge usually occurs when goals have been achieved. The patient needs to be involved with his/her discharge planning in order for discharge to be successful. The following topics need to be included in the discharge plan: major goals or problems, services received by the patient, the patient's response to the intervention or services, received condition of patient when discharged, specific referrals/information or instructions given to the patient or patient's family.

When charting, it is important to know the various charting symbols, any accepted descriptive words, and exactly how to chart. The following is a modified list of charting guidelines:

- Write legibly.
- Always use a black pen, never a pencil.
- Don't tamper with the record, e.g., change the sequence of the notes.
- If an error was made, draw a single line through the error and then date and initial it.
- Do not vent anger or frustration with the family or patient in the chart.
- Document services provided and document if services are refused.
- Document any incidents.
- Sign and date every entry.

Remember, generally speaking, if you are unsure about whether or not to document something, if it is not documented, it did not happen. (Austin, 2004; Burlingame & Blaschko, 2002; Shank & Coyle, 2002; Stumbo & Peterson, 2004; Sylvester, Voelkl, & Ellis, 2001; Wilhite & Keller, 2000).

Documentation procedures for program accountability and payment for services is the second competency in Documentation and Evaluation. According to Stumbo and Peterson (2004), "…. Accurate and complete documentation [is necessary] in order to 1) assure the delivery of quality services, 2) facilitate communication among staff, 3) provide for professional accountability, 4) comply with administrative requirements and 5) provide data for quality improvement and efficacy research" (p. 316). Therapeutic recreation specialists, like other professionals, are accountable for

services rendered and outcomes achieved. Accurate documentation can provide the necessary evidence.

The type of documentation required is set by the agency in which the therapeutic recreation specialist works. Accrediting agencies like JCAHO and CARF have standards that impact documentation. The Centers for Medicare and Medicaid Services (CMS) require documentation to indicate that services were necessary. The CMS requires that the staff complete the *Minimum Data Set for Resident Assessment and Care Screening* (MDS) which includes a section on activity pursuit patterns. Therapeutic recreation specialists may also be required to complete Section T of the MDS when therapeutic recreation services are ordered by a physician. Based on the information from the MDS the Resident Assessment Protocol Summary (RAPS) may be completed. Third-party payers are interested in documentation because it is from this information they will make decisions about reimbursement. Thus, it is very important that the therapeutic recreation specialist is very clear when writing problems, goals, and interventions used, and responses of the patient to those interventions (Austin, 2004; Shank & Coyle, 2002; Stumbo & Peterson, 2004).

The third competency is *Methods for interpretation of progress notes, observations, and assessment results of the person served.* It is very important that the therapeutic recreation specialist be able to interpret the medical chart. One needs to understand the doctor's orders, the assessments/notes from other disciplines, and be able to interpret their meaning. Very often it is not necessary for a therapeutic recreation specialist to assess a patient in a certain area if it has already been thoroughly assessed by another discipline. It is necessary for the therapeutic recreation specialist to understand what has been stated by the other discipline and use that information when developing a treatment plan.

The fourth competency in Documentation and Evaluation is *Methods for evaluating agency/TR service programs*. This subtopic ensures that the entry-level professional understands a variety of evaluation methods. A therapeutic recreation department must determine what is important—what should be evaluated. Usually it is determined that quality of services delivered, effectiveness of those programs, and the outcomes of those programs are of most interest to the department, the agency, third-party payers, and the receiver of services. So how is evaluation conducted? First, one must differentiate between formative and summative evaluation. When evaluation is formative, it is ongoing and occurs while the program is in progress. Staff can make changes on a daily or weekly basis dependent on what the evaluation data indicates. Summative evaluation is conducted at the end of a program and can be used to compare programs or provide information for the next session of programming. For summative evaluation, the program is completely finished when the data is collected and analyzed. It is also necessary to understand the importance of an evaluation plan and the need to develop specific data-collection instruments. According to Stumbo and Peterson (2004), there are several ways to collect evaluation data: using questionnaires, by observation, or by record documentation (p. 369).

The need to establish an administrative schedule for evaluation and determine the program revision process following data collection is a task for the therapeutic recreation specialist (Riley, 1987; Stumbo & Peterson, 2004; Sylvester, Voelkl, & Ellis, 2001).

The last subtopic in this knowledge area is *methods for quality improvement/performance improvement*. This is the most common method of evaluating therapeutic recreation services and is mandated by external accreditation agencies. Quality improvement is not just one activity but a variety of activities that provide useful data on the quality of care for patients. According to Stumbo and Peterson, a basic approach to "comprehensive service evaluation involves a . . .process that focuses on a) seeking out problematic areas that lower quality, b) correcting those problems, and c) evaluating how well those corrections are solving the problems" (pp. 388-389). The therapeutic recreation specialist needs to understand and be able to design an effective evaluation plan, focusing on identifying important aspects of care (i.e., client assessment, treatment plans, specific intervention techniques used, patient safety or risk management, staff training and continuing education, etc.). After identifying the aspects of care on which the evaluation will be focused, the therapeutic recreation specialist identifies how to collect the data, collects the data, analyzes the data, and then makes the identified changes in patient care (McCormick, 2003; Riley, 1987; Riley, 1991; Stumbo & Peterson, 2004; Sylvester, Voelkl, & Ellis, 2001).

Information related to this knowledge area is usually covered in junior and senior level therapeutic recreation courses that relate directly to programming, since documentation and evaluation are important components of therapeutic recreation treatment. While they are not included in this *Study Guide*, nor mentioned in the competencies, therapeutic recreation specialists are expected to understand medical terminology and documentation terms. Information on quality improvement and evaluation also may be found in some therapeutic recreation administration and management courses.

References Related to Documentation and Evaluation

Austin, D. R. (2004). *Therapeutic recreation: Processes and techniques* (5th ed.). Champaign, IL: Sagamore Publishing.

Burlingame, J., & Blaschko, T. M. (2002). *Assessment tools for recreational therapy* (3rd ed.). Ravensdale, WA: Idyll Arbor.

McCormick, B. P. (2003). Outcome measurement as a tool for performance improvement. In N. J. Stumbo (Ed.), *Client outcomes in therapeutic recreation* (pp. 221-232). State College, PA: Venture Publishing.

Riley, B. (Ed.). (1987). *Evaluation of therapeutic recreation through quality assurance.* State College, PA: Venture Publishing.

Riley, B. (Ed.). (1991). *Quality management: Applications for therapeutic recreation.* State College, PA: Venture Publishing.

Shank J., & Coyle, C. (2002). *Therapeutic recreation in health promotion and rehabilitation.* State College, PA: Venture Publishing.

Stumbo, N. J., & Peterson, C. A. (2003). *Therapeutic recreation program design: Principles and procedures* (4th ed.). San Francisco, CA: Pearson.

Sylvester, C., Voelkl, J. E., & Ellis, G. D. (2001). *Therapeutic recreation programming: Theory and practice.* State College, PA: Venture Publishing.

Wilhite, B. C., & Keller, M. J. (2000). *Therapeutic recreation: Cases and exercises* (2nd ed.). State College, PA: Venture Publishing.

Organizing and Managing Services

Most entry-level professionals are not solely responsible for the organization and management of a therapeutic recreation department. However, there are many therapists who are one person departments and therefore need to understand some basic organization and management principles and requirements. In addition, even if this is not a direct job function, all specialists, regardless of job held, need an understanding of the organization and management functions. Thus, this knowledge area will provide approximately 9% or eight questions. There are seven competencies that relate to *Organizing and Managing Services:* Components of an Agency/TR Service Plan of Operation; Personnel, Intern, and Volunteer Supervision and Management; Budgeting and Fiscal Responsibility for Service Delivery; Area and Facility Management; Quality Improvement; Payment Systems; and Accreditation Standards and Regulations.

The first competency, *Components of an Agency/TR Service Plan of Operation,* relates to the development of a plan of operation or how the agency or therapeutic recreation services operate. For some organizations, specifically in the community, this will be known as a policy and procedures manual. For most health care organizations, the policy and procedures manual is contained within the Plan of Operation. There are two plans of operation with which the therapeutic recreation specialist should be concerned: 1) the agency's plan of operation, and 2) the therapeutic recreation department's plan of operation.

The agency's plan of operation should adequately include therapeutic recreation services as a component of service. Accreditation surveyors will review thoroughly the overall agency's plan of operation, including services provided by therapeutic recreation specialists. The agency plan of operation should include patient management functions and program management functions, with therapeutic recreation included as appropriate. Examples of patient management functions include client assessment, treatment plans, progress notes, treatment plan reviews, and discharge summaries. Examples of program management functions include a quality improvement process, utilizations reviews, and patient care monitoring procedures.

Every therapeutic recreation department or unit needs to have a written plan of operation. All staff should be familiar with this document and utilize its procedures. The therapeutic recreation department's or unit's plan of operation should have a written philosophy that reflects the philosophy of the agency, have overall goals for the program, and describe the purpose and function of therapeutic recreation within the agency. It also should have information regarding the nature and diversity of activities to be utilized with clients and include information related to both patient management functions and program management functions. Examples of patient management functions within the therapeutic recreation department's plan of operation include the client assessment process, treatment plans, interventions used, discharge planning, etc. Examples of program management functions within the therapeutic recreation plan of operation include staff organization and development, quality improvement, utilization review, patient care monitoring, etc. A plan of operation is a requirement for a department and is part of the standards of practice for both national organizations (American Therapeutic Recreation Association, 1991; National Therapeutic Recreation Society, 1994; Navar & Dunn, 1981; O'Morrow & Carter, 1997; Riley, 1987, 1991; Stumbo & Peterson, 2003).

The second competency relates to *Personnel, intern, and volunteer supervision and management.* This section focuses on the need for some entry-level therapeutic recre-

ation specialists to be able to supervise a variety of people. Primarily it focuses on the supervision of staff, volunteers, and student interns.

The supervision of other therapists is referred to as "clinical supervision." According to Austin (2004), there are two purposes of clinical supervision: 1) to improve clinical practice skills, and 2) to ensure that the therapeutic intents of a program are being provided or met. The three roles a clinical supervisor may perform include teacher, counselor and consultant. The supervisor and supervisee together establish goals that the supervisee wishes to attain. Based on those goals, the content of the supervision program and a time frame is established. The last step is evaluation. As an entry-level practitioner, you are not expected to provide clinical supervision at this point in your career; but, a quality clinical supervision program will help you grow and expand your ability to deliver quality services.

Volunteers play an important role in many therapeutic recreation departments, and many entry-level practitioners need to be able to supervise them. It is important that when a department determines it has a need for volunteers, that the department establishes a volunteer plan including policies, job descriptions, and a marketing plan with promotional materials for recruitment and retention. It is important that program guidelines be established and that while volunteers may be used for parts of the program, they may not be used for the implementation of an intervention. For example, volunteers may be used to provide animals for an animal-assisted therapy program, but it is the therapeutic recreation specialist who is responsible for the assessment, development of the goals for the program, and the therapeutic use of the animals. Many long-term care facilities use volunteers to "call" *Bingo*™ but if the therapist is using *Bingo*™ as a therapeutic activity, it is up to the therapeutic recreation specialist to determine if the patient's objectives were met and to document the intervention process.

The supervision of interns is another important role of a therapeutic recreation specialist. It is not expected that an entry-level therapeutic recreation specialist would be supervising an intern. However, in preparation for an intern, a department should identify internship goals and objectives, establish policies and procedures, ensure the staff and facility are prepared to accept interns, develop training materials, establish an intern manual, determine selection procedures, and establish a recruitment plan. According to O'Morrow and Carter (1997), there are three major tasks that an intern supervisor needs to provide: communication with and observation of the intern, documentation of intern activities and experiences, and provision of training and education opportunities.

The third competency of Organizing and Managing Services relates to *Budgeting and fiscal responsibility for service delivery*. This competency expects the entry-level professional to have some understanding of fiscal matters. There are a variety of sources from which therapeutic recreation services may receive funding. These revenue sources include tax based appropriations from the federal, state, or local government; grants and contracts; contributions and donations; fees, charges and reimbursement; and a combination of any of the aforementioned sources. It is important for the entry-level therapist to understand the source of program revenue. Most community programs revenue sources are tax-based appropriations and fees for services. Within health care facilities, most consumers are charged directly

for services and these charges may be paid by insurance companies or third-party payers. Therapeutic recreation services are considered either ancillary services or routine services. Ancillary services are usually prescribed by a physician to meet a consumer need. Routine services are those provided as a part of basic services and are usually built into the overhead or operating costs.

There are different types of budgets used in therapeutic recreation services. The first kind of budget is a "revenue and expense" or "operating" budget. This type of budget delineates the day-to-day expenses and revenues for a year. A "capital expenditure" budget is related to long range planning and usually spans a three- to five-year period. A "program" budget is focused on meeting goals and objectives or allocating resources based on costs and benefits of specific programs. "Zero-based" budgeting requires that a manager is re-evaluating the programs within their department annually. Every program must be rejustified, and just because a program was funded one year at a certain level does not mean it will be again. A manager using zero-based budgeting is forced to set priorities and justify resources annually. Lastly, a "flexible" budget allows a manager to adjust a budget dependent upon unexpected occurrences like a smaller number of patients or patients who are more severely injured and require different, perhaps more intense, interventions than previously budgeted (cf., O'Morrow & Carter, 1997).

Frequently therapeutic recreation specialists are responsible for *Area and facility management* which is the fourth competency in this Knowledge area. It is important to understand how the areas and facilities are going to be used. A therapeutic recreation specialist needs to have a good understanding of accessibility standards and requirements for specific recreation areas such as trails or playgrounds or pools. A risk management plan for each area and facility for which the therapeutic recreation specialist is in charge is important to develop. A risk management plan will evaluate the amount of risk that an area or piece of equipment may present and establishes policies and procedures that staff must follow in order to reduce risk.

Quality (Performance) Improvement (QI or PI) is the fifth competency in this knowledge area. Although quality improvement has been addressed earlier, this competency has some subtopics. Also, quality improvement is now referred to as *performance improvement*. The first portion of performance improvement that is addressed through this competency is utilization review. *Utilization review* refers to looking at how effectively a department uses it's resources. Utilization review addresses over-utilization, under-utilization, and inefficiency. This is a program management function that should be in a written plan of operation for a health care agency.

Risk management plans are an important part of all therapeutic recreation services. Every department needs to develop risk management plans for all of their service areas and programs. Essentially, what a risk management plan does is to identify all potential risks that could occur in a facility, with equipment or during a program to an employee, patient or family member. Then, the therapeutic recreation specialist develops a plan that will eliminate, reduce, or manage that risk. It involves loss prevention and control, and handling all incidents, claims and other insurance, or litigation-related tasks (Stumbo & Peterson, 2004, p. 491).

The last subtopic under *Quality (Performance) Improvement* is the important area of outcome monitoring. In short, "outcomes" are the differences that occur in a person from when they begin treatment or enter the health care facility to when they leave treatment or

the health care facility. Of course, it is hoped that these changes will be positive. Currently outcome measurement is being discussed rather than outcome monitoring. JCAHO (as cited in McCormick, 2003) has identified three categories of outcome measures: health status (functional well being of an individual), patient perceptions of care (satisfaction measures of care from patient or family perspective), and clinical performance outcomes (outcomes of processes of care). Therapeutic recreation specialists need to understand outcomes and be able to support positive outcomes as a result of their treatment. This will entail some efficacy research. According to Stumbo and Peterson (2004), "efficacy is the improvement in health outcome achieved in a research setting, in expert hands, under ideal circumstances" (p. 487). This research is usually done to determine the effectiveness of an intervention with a particular diagnosis (JCAHO, 1999; McCormick, 2003; Stumbo & Peterson, 2004).

The sixth competency in Organizing and Managing Services is *Payment systems (e.g., managed care, PPO, private contract, Medicare, Medicaid)*. After years of using the retrospective payment system in health care organizations, managed care systems are now the predominant payment method. Managed care systems have shifted the authority of determining the services the patient needs from the providers of care to the payers for care. Therapeutic recreation specialists are always challenged by the insurance companies regarding the need for their services (Shank & Coyle, 2002). According to Thompson (2001), the prospective payment system (PPS) has the following elements: "1) It is a price-based system; 2) Prices are set in advance; 3) The price is inclusive of all services provided; 4) No additional payment or settlement will occur; and 5) The current year's actual costs do not impact the price established" (p. 252). The

PPS was established to contain health care costs, ensure quality, assure Medicare recipients access to care, and it has a beneficiary-centered focus. Medicare is a federal health insurance program that provides care for people 65 and over, for people with certain disabilities, and people with end-stage renal disease. The program has two parts: part A provides for hospital care, skilled nursing care, home health care, and hospice services; while, part B provides supplemental medical insurance. It covers physician services, outpatient services, emergency department visits, and medical equipment. Medicaid is a combined program of state and federal insurance for qualified needy individuals. When finances have been depleted by medical care, Medicaid will pay the difference between income and cost of care (Carter, van Andel, & Robb, 2003; McCormick, 2002; O'Morrow & Carter, 1997; Shank & Coyle, 2002; Skalko, 1998; Stumbo & Peterson, 2004; Thompson, 2001).

The last subtopic relates to *Accreditation standards and regulations.* This subtopic ensures that the entry-level professional has a working knowledge of the accrediting bodies and their regulations. The Centers for Medicare and Medicaid Services (CMS), is responsible for establishing regulations for both Medicare and Medicaid. CMS was formerly the Health Care Financing Administration. It is important to keep track of the regulations established by CMS if you have patients who are receiving funding from Medicare or Medicaid. The Joint Commission on Accreditation of Healthcare Organizations (JCAHO) accredits a variety of hospitals and facilities. The Rehabilitation Accreditation Commission (CARF) also mandates standards that relate directly to the provision of therapeutic recreation services. In fact CARF requires that a certified therapeutic recreation specialist be provided for all in-patient rehabil-

itation services (Carter, van Andel, & Robb, 2003; Shank & Coyle, 2002; Stumbo & Peterson, 2004).

Information for this section can be found in administration of therapeutic recreation or organization and management of therapeutic recreation coursework. Some topics may be covered in issues in therapeutic recreation courses.

References Related to Organizing and Managing Services

American Therapeutic Recreation Association. (2001). *Standards for the practice of therapeutic recreation and self-assessment guide.* Alexandria, VA: Author.

Austin, D. R. (2004). *Therapeutic recreation: Processes and techniques* (5th ed.). Champaign, IL: Sagamore Publishing.

Carter, M. J., van Andel, G. E., & Robb, G. M. (2003). *Therapeutic recreation: A practical approach* (3rd ed.). Prospect Heights, IL: Waveland Press.

McCormick, B. P. (2002). Healthcare in America: An overview. In D. R. Austin, J. Dattilo, & B. P. McCormick (Eds.), *Conceptual foundations for therapeutic recreation* (pp. 185-206). State College, PA: Venture Publishing.

McCormick, B. P. (2003). Outcomes measurement as a tool for performance improvement. In N. J. Stumbo (Ed.), *Client outcomes in therapeutic recreation services: On competence and outcomes* (pp. 221-231). Champaign, IL: Sagamore Publishing.

National Therapeutic Recreation Society. (1994). *Standards of practice for therapeutic recreation services.* Alexandria, VA: National Recreation and Park Association.

Navar, N., & Dunn, J. (Eds.). (1981). *Quality assurance: Concerns for therapeutic recreation.* Urbana-Champaign, IL: University of Illinois.

O'Morrow, G. S., & Carter, M. J.(1997). *Effective management in therapeutic recreation service.* State College, PA: Venture Publishing.

Riley, B. (Ed.). (1987). *Evaluation of therapeutic recreation through quality assurance.* State College, PA: Venture Publishing.

Riley, B. (Ed.). (1991). *Quality management: Applications for therapeutic recreation.* State College, PA: Venture Publishing.

Shank, J., & Coyle, C. (2002). *Therapeutic recreation in health promotion and rehabilitation.* State College, PA: Venture Publishing.

Skalko, T. (1998) Reimbursement. In F. Brasile, T. K. Skalko, & J. Burlingame (Eds.), *Perspectives in recreational therapy* (pp. 447-462). Ravensdale, WA: Idyll Arbor.

Stumbo, N. J. (2003). Outcomes, accountability, and therapeutic recreation. In N. J. Stumbo (Ed.), *Client outcomes in therapeutic recreation services: On competence and outcomes* (pp. 1-24). Champaign, IL: Sagamore Publishing.

Stumbo, N. J., & Peterson, C. A. (2004) *Therapeutic recreation program design: Principles and procedures.* San Francisco, CA: Benjamin Cummings.

Thompson, G. T. (2001) Reimbursement: Surviving prospective payment as a recreational therapy practitioner. In N. J. Stumbo (Ed.), *Professional issues in therapeutic recreation: On competence and outcomes* (pp. 249-264). Champaign, IL: Sagamore Publishing.

Advancement of the Profession

The last knowledge area relates to *Advancement of the profession.* Seven percent of the test comes from this area. This knowledge area contains the following competencies: Professionalism; Requirements for TR certification/recertification; Advocacy for persons served; Legislation and regulations pertaining to TR; Professional standards and ethical guidelines pertaining to TR; Public relations, promotion, and marketing of the TR profession; Methods, resources, and references for maintaining and upgrading professional competencies; Knowledge of professional associations and organizations; and Interactive process among pre-services, in-service, and direct service for the advancement of the profession. Many of these competencies have been covered in previous knowledge areas.

The first competency relates to *Professionalism: Guidelines for the development of the profession.* This competency suggests that the entry-level professional know what a profession is, what the qualities of a profession are, and what it means to be a professional. It is recommended that the entry-level professional have an understanding of the roots of the therapeutic recreation profession, especially the formation of the early organizations (e.g., Hospital Recreation Society, Recreation Therapy Section, National Association for Recreational Therapists, and CAHR), and the development of the current professional societies (see the first knowledge area Background for the development of professional societies).

Austin (2002) suggests there are nine qualities that help define professionalism. The first is an appropriate educational background, meaning that you should have received a degree in therapeutic recreation or recreation with an emphasis in therapeutic recreation with the appropriate quantity and quality of coursework that prepares you to work in the field. Following graduation, you should feel like you are ready to practice. Second, you should have a professional organization as your major reference. In other words, whether you choose the American Therapeutic Recreation Association or the National Therapeutic Recreation Society you need to have one to which you can turn when you have problems or questions. You should attend conferences and read literature from that organization to keep you up-to-date on trends and issues within the field. The third quality a professional has is the individual beliefs in autonomy and self-regulation. The person follows a specific code of ethics and standard of practice. They believe they can make their own professional judgments. Fourth, you should believe in the value of your profession. Do you believe that therapeutic recreation is important, and do you behave in a way that demonstrates that belief by advocating for the profession? The fifth quality relates to having a calling to the profession. Do you believe that this is something you just have to do; you truly believe that therapeutic recreation is something that you have been drawn to and you must work in the field to be satisfied? The fifth quality is contributing to the body of knowledge. Whether it is participating in research, writing an article for a newsletter or a book, a professional makes contributions to the body of knowledge. Providing professional and community service is the sixth quality. A professional takes an active role in a professional organization, whether it is at the local or national level and also works to improve services in the community for people with disabilities. The seventh quality states that a professional will continue to grow and learn by attending conferences or reading professional journals. And the last quality relates to theory-based practice. Every professional should follow the therapeutic recreation process, accept and follow a practice model and continue to read and incorporate techniques that have been researched and accepted as an appropriate intervention technique (Austin, 2002;

Carter, van Andel, & Robb, 2003; Kraus & Shank, 1992).

The entry-level professional needs to understand the *requirements for TR certification and recertification requirements*. There are two paths to certification; the first and most common path is the academic path. To qualify for the academic path, an individual must have a major in therapeutic recreation or a major in recreation with an option in therapeutic recreation. The major in therapeutic recreation must contain a minimum of 18 semester hours (for this section all hours are calculated to semester hours—for quarter-hours please go to the NCTRC website) of therapeutic recreation and general recreation content coursework with no less than nine semester hours in therapeutic recreation content. There must be support coursework totaling 18 semester hours including three hours of course work in anatomy and physiology; three hours in abnormal psychology and three hours in human growth and development across the lifespan. And, there must be a minimum of 480 hours, 12 consecutive weeks of field placement (internship) under a certified therapeutic recreation specialist (NCTRC, 2004).

The second path to certification is through the equivalency path. There are two (2) equivalency paths to certification. Like the academic path, all individuals must take 18 semester hours in therapeutic recreation and general recreation course work. The supportive coursework requirements are different dependent upon whether the person takes equivalency path A or B. Under the equivalency path, full-time paid work experience can be substituted for the field placement requirement. Please visit the NCTRC website (www.NCTRC.org) for the equivalency standards.

After submitting the transcripts to NCTRC and the application to sit for the exam, the applicant will be notified whether he is eligible to sit for the exam. If there is an error or the individual is not eligible, the applicant may appeal. If the applicant meets the standards, he will be notified that he may sit for the exam.

The test is a 90-item computer-based test, and you have 86 minutes to complete it. When you have completed the test you will receive a) notification that you have passed the test, b) notification that you have failed the test, or c) notification that your score falls in a range where you have neither passed or failed and you will be given 15 more questions until the computer is able to determine a passing or failing score. The additional questions are referred to as "testlets."

Annual renewal and recertification are two important processes a therapeutic recreation specialist must be aware of. The certification cycle is five years in length. Each year of that cycle the certified individual must submit an annual maintenance application and fee. There are two different options from which a certified person can choose in order to become recertified. The first option consists of a combination of professional experience and continuing education; the second option is simply retaking and passing the national exam. Please visit the NCTRC website (www.NCTRC.org) for information regarding what opportunities are available for continuing education.

A therapeutic recreation specialist is expected to provide *Advocacy*. A good advocate is one who continues to help people get their needs met and if that means continuous education, then you must be prepared to do so. One of the other roles of a therapeutic recreation specialist is to act as an "advocate" for a client. To advocate means to recommend or plead for a specific cause or policy and speak on behalf of another. Very often, it is up to the therapeutic recreation specialist to advo-cate for recreation services for specific clients/patients especially when they return to the community. They may also advocate for clients'/patients' specific needs in treatment team meetings to ensure that a client/patient receive the treatment or equipment that he or she requires. Another kind of advocacy that a professional is expected to do is to advocate for their profession. Whether it is advocating for legislative recognition or recognition by the treatment team regarding the importance of therapeutic recreation, the professional must be willing to speak up in support of his or her profession (Austin, 2002; Bullock & Mahon, 2001; Carter & LeConey, 2004; Dattilo, 2002).

Legislation and regulations pertaining to therapeutic recreation has been well covered in the knowledge area, Planning the Intervention. However, one initiative was not previously mentioned that should involve therapeutic recreation specialists. That initiative is *Healthy People 2010*. Focus area six specifically speaks to *Disability and Secondary Conditions*. The Healthy People initiative is a 10-year plan that intends to "...encourage and guide federal, state, local, private, and community health promotion and wellness activities and policies to improve the health of Americans" (NCBDDD, 2002, p. 1). Therapeutic recreation specialists need to be aware of this initiative and work within their community to support and assist in the improvement of the health and well-being of persons with disabilities (NCBDDD, 2002).

It is important that entry-level professionals be aware of the *Professional Standards and Ethical Guidelines* which pertain to Therapeutic Recreation. The professional needs to understand and utilize the Standards of Practice from both the American Therapeutic Recreation Association (ATRA) and the National Therapeutic Recreation Society (NTRS). Both organizations have developed Codes of Ethics and those guidelines should be understood. Both the Codes of Ethics and the Standards of Practice were reviewed in the knowledge area of Planning the Intervention. The National Therapeutic Recreation Society also provides *Guidelines for the Administration of Therapeutic Recreation Services.*

The National Council for Therapeutic Recreation Certification (NCTRC) is responsible for standards for the certification of therapeutic recreation personnel. It is also responsible for placing sanctions on any individual who has violated any NCTRC Certification Standards or any other NCTRC standard, policy, or procedure.

The Council on Accreditation is responsible for the revision and administration of the standards for the accreditation of recreation education programs in colleges and universities. It is also responsible for the creation and administration of the standards for the therapeutic recreation option. (ATRA, 1991, 2001; NCTRC, 2004; NTRS, 1990, 1994).

If the profession is to continue, it is very important that every professional be involved in *public relations, promotion, and marketing* of the therapeutic recreation profession. This competency is instrumental in ensuring that therapeutic recreation has a part in the health care arena. Very often therapeutic recreation services can be marketed using the "value added" approach. Thus, the addition of or continued use of therapeutic recreation services will improve quality of care for a health care agency. It is important to be able to promote and market therapeutic recreation at the local, state, and national level to legislators, health care providers, and third-party payers. It is also important to be able to market therapeutic recreation to other health care providers especially physicians and members of the treatment team (Carter, van Andel, & Robb, 2003; O'Morrow & Carter, 1997).

The seventh competency relates to *Methods, resources and references for maintaining and upgrading professional competencies.* This competency expects the entry-level professional to understand the importance of continuing education. In order to maintain certification, the therapeutic recreation specialist must demonstrate his willingness to participate in continuing education opportunities. NCTRC recognizes a variety of methods that a person can utilize in order to receive continuing education units (CEUs), each method the person chooses must relate to one of the NCTRC Job Analysis Knowledge areas. These methods include: taking courses for academic credit; attending therapeutic recreation continuing education programs at conferences and workshops, writing publications; making presentations at seminars and conferences or presenting guest lectures in courses; and making poster presentations.

The American Therapeutic Recreation Association has developed a series of methods for continuing education, all presented under the ATRA Academy. It acknowledges that continuing education is important to all professionals, and formal education through colleges and universities is not the only way to attain educational competencies. It provides a variety of methods to receive CEUs.

The National Therapeutic Recreation Society also offers continuing education units through its national conference. A person can also receive CEUs by contributing to the *Therapeutic Recreation Journal.*

The eighth competency in *Advancement of the Profession* relates to *Knowledge of professional associations and organizations.* The entry-level professional needs to be aware of the national professional associations in therapeutic recreation: the National Therapeutic Recreation Society and the American Therapeutic Recreation Association. It is a good idea to understand under what circumstances each was formed and the purposes/goals of each organization. There are state and local organizations that also play a role in the profession. The entry-level professional needs to understand the purposes of these important associations. It is vital to understand that NCTRC is not a professional organization but a certifying body, thus differing from both ATRA and NTRS in goals, purpose, activities, and membership. The history of these organizations can be found in the knowledge area of Background. More information on the services these professional organizations and our credentialing organization provide can be found on their web sites.

American Therapeutic Recreation Association: www.atra-tr.org

National Therapeutic Recreation Society: www.nrpa.org. Click on branches and sections, then click on National Therapeutic Recreation Society.

National Council for Therapeutic Recreation Certification: www.nctrc.org

The Role of Interactive process among pre-services, in-service, and direct service for the advancement of the TR profession (e.g., internships, collaborative research, presentations) is the last competency in Advancement of the Profession. As the saying goes, "It takes a village to raise a child," and it certainly takes a community of people collaborating to make a strong profession. The profession expects collaboration between practitioners and educators in internships, research, presentations at conferences, and the authoring of articles and books. Together these professionals can develop and promote a healthy and strong profession.

Information about *Advancement of the Profession* can be found in many therapeutic recreation courses. Usually information is found in introductory classes, senior seminar classes, or professional issues classes.

References Related to Advancement of the Profession

American Therapeutic Recreation Association. (1990). *Code of ethics.* Alexandria, VA: Author.

American Therapeutic Recreation Association. (1998). *Finding the path: Ethics in action.* Hattiesburg, MS: Author.

American Therapeutic Recreation Association. (1991). *Standards for the practice of therapeutic recreation.* Alexandria, VA: Author.

American Therapeutic Recreation Association. (2000). *Standards for the practice of therapeutic recreation and self assessment guide* (2nd ed.). Alexandria, VA: Author..

Austin, D. R. (2002). Professionalism. In D. R. Austin, J. Dattilo, & B. P. McCormick (Eds.), *Conceptual foundations for therapeutic recreation* (pp. 265-271). State College, PA: Venture Publishing.

Austin, D. R. (2004). *Therapeutic recreation: Processes and techniques* (5th ed.). Champaign, IL: Sagamore Publishing.

Brasile, F., Skalko, T. K., & Burlingame, J. (1998). *Perspectives in recreational therapy.* Ravensdale, WA: Idyll Arbor.

Bullock, C. C., & Mahon, M. J. (2001). *Introduction to recreation services for people with disabilities: A person-centered approach.* Champaign, IL: Sagamore Publishing.

Carter, M. J., & LeConey, S. P. (2004). *Therapeutic recreation in the community: An inclusive approach* (2nd ed.). Champaign, IL: Sagamore Publishing.

Carter, M. J., van Andel, G. E., & Robb, G. M. (2003). *Therapeutic recreation: A practical approach* (3rd ed.). Prospect Heights, IL: Waveland Press.

Dattilo, J. (2002). *Inclusive leisure services: Responding to the rights of people with disabilities* (2nd ed.). State College, PA: Venture Publishing.

Kraus, R., & Shank, J. (1992). *Therapeutic recreation service: Principles and practices* (4th ed.). Dubuque, IA: Wm. C. Brown.

National Center on Birth Defects and Developmental Disabilities. (2002). *Healthy people with disabilities: State information* [Brochure]. Atlanta, GA: Center for Disease Control and Prevention.

National Council for Therapeutic Recreation Certification. (2004). *Candidate Bulletin* [Electronic Version]. Thiells, NY: Author.

National Therapeutic Recreation Society. (1994). *Standards of practice for therapeutic recreation services.* Arlington, VA: Author.

National Therapeutic Recreation Society. (1990a). *Code of ethics and interpretive guidelines.* Arlington, VA: Author.

National Therapeutic Recreation Society. (1990b). *Guidelines for the administration of therapeutic recreation services.* Arlington, VA: Author.

National Therapeutic Recreation Society. (2003). *Standards of practice for therapeutic recreation services and annotated bibliography.* Arlington, VA: Author

O'Morrow, J. S., & Carter, M. J. (1997). *Effective management in therapeutic recreation services.* State College, PA: Venture Publishing.

Shank, J., & Coyle, C. (2002). *Therapeutic recreation in health promotion and rehabilitation.* State College, PA: Venture Publishing.

The following is a list of textbooks and references used in therapeutic recreation. It is not all inclusive; however, it may assist you when searching for a reference to learn more about a specific topic.

Therapeutic Recreation Literature Textbooks

American Therapeutic Recreation Association. (1998). *Finding the path: Ethics in action.* Hattiesburg, MS: Author. ISBN 1-889435-13-9

American Therapeutic Recreation Association. (2000). *Standards for the practice of therapeutic recreation and self-assessment guide* (2nd ed.). Alexandria, VA: Author. ISBN 1-889435-02-3

Armstrong, M., & Lauzen, S. (1994) *Community integration program.* Ravensdale, WA: Idyll Arbor. ISBN 1-882883-09-8

Austin, D. R. (2004). *Therapeutic recreation: Processes and techniques* (5th ed.). Champaign, IL: Sagamore Publishing. ISBN 1-57167-524-8

Austin, D. R. (2001). *Glossary of recreation therapy and occupational therapy.* State College, PA: Venture Publishing. ISBN 1-892132-19-2

Austin, D. R., & Crawford, M. E. (1996). *Therapeutic recreation: An introduction* (2nd ed.). Needham Heights, MA: Allyn & Bacon. ISBN 0-13-110736-4

Austin, D. R., Dattilo, J., & McCormick, B. P. (2002). *Conceptual foundations for therapeutic recreation.* State College, PA: Venture Publishing, Inc. ISBN 1-892132-30-3

Avedon, E. M. (1974). *Therapeutic recreation: An applied behavioral science approach.* Englewood Cliffs, NJ: Prentice-Hall, Inc. ISBN 0-3-914879-5

Baglin, C. A., Lewis, M. E. B., & Williams, B. (2004). *Recreation and leisure for persons with emotional problems and challenging behaviors.* Champaign, IL: Sagamore Publishing. ISBN 1-57167-521-3

Bender, M., & Baglin, C. A. (2004). *Implementing recreation and leisure opportunities for infants and toddlers with disabilities.*

Champaign, IL: Sagamore Publishing. ISBN 1-57167-384-9

Bender, M., Brannan, S. A., & Verhoven, P. J. (1984). *Leisure education for the handicapped: Curriculum, goals, activities and resources.* San Diego, CA: College Hill Press, Inc. ISBN 0-933014-10-4

Boothman, S. (2002). *Measurable assessment in recreation for resident-centered care.* High Rolls Mtn. Park, NM: Sienna's Mark. No ISBN.

Brannon, S., Fullerton, A., Arick, J., Robb, G., & Bender, M. (2004). *Including youth with disabilities in outdoor programs: Best practices, outcomes, and resources.* Champaign, IL: Sagamore Publishing. ISBN 1-57167-500-0

Brasile, F., Skalko, T. K., & Burlingame, J. (1998). *Perspectives in recreational therapy.* Ravensdale, WA: Idyll Arbor. ISBN 1-882883-26-8

Buettner, L., & Fitzsimmons, S. (2003). *Dementia practice guideline for recreational therapy: Treatment of disturbing behaviors.* Alexandria, VA: American Therapeutic Recreation Association. ISBN 1-889435-22-8

Buettner, L., & Martin, S. (1995). *Therapeutic recreation in the nursing home.* State College, PA: Venture Publishing. ISBN 0-910251-76-2

Bullock, C. C., & Mahon, M. J. (2001). *Introduction to recreation services for people with disabilities: A person-centered approach.* Champaign, IL: Sagamore Publishing. ISBN 1-57167-381-4

Burlingame, J., & Blaschko, T. (2002). *Assessment tools for recreational therapy and related fields* (3rd ed.). Ravensdale, WA: Idyll Arbor. ISBN 1-882883-45-4

Burlingame, J. (2001). *Idyll Arbor's therapy dictionary.* Ravensdale, WA: Idyll Arbor. ISBN 1-882883-46-2

Carter, M. J. (1991). *Designing therapeutic recreation programs in the community.* Reston, VA: American Alliance for Health, Physical Education, Recreation and Dance. ISBN 0-88314-518-9

Carter, M. J., & Leconey, S. P. (2004). *Therapeutic recreation in the community: An inclusive approach* (2nd ed.). Champaign, IL: Sagamore Publishing. ISBN 1-57167-513-2

Carter, M. J., van Andel, G. E., & Robb, G. M. (2003). *Therapeutic recreation: A practical approach* (3rd ed.). Prospect Heights, IL: Waveland Press. ISBN 1-57766-219-9

Compton, D. M. (Ed.). (1989). *Issues in therapeutic recreation: A profession in transition.* Champaign, IL: Sagamore Publishing. ISBN 0-915611-20-1

Compton, D. M. (Ed.). (1997). *Issues in therapeutic recreation: Toward the new millennium* (2nd ed.). Champaign, IL: Sagamore Publishing. ISBN 1-57167-031-9

Compton D. M., & Iso-Ahola, S. E. (Eds.). (1994). *Leisure and mental health.* Ravensdale, WA: Idyll Arbor. ISBN 0-934309-86-8

Coyle, C. P., Kinney, W. B., Riley, B., & Shank, J. W. (1991). *Benefits of therapeutic recreation: A consensus view.* Ravensdale, WA: Idyll Arbor. ISBN 1-882883-06-3

Coyne, P., & Fullerton, A. (2004). *Supporting individuals with autism spectrum disorder in recreation.* Champaign, IL: Sagamore Publishing. ISBN 1-57167-498-5

Crawford, M. E., & Mendell, R. (1987). *Therapeutic recreation and adapted physical activities for mentally retarded individuals.* Englewood Cliffs, NJ: Prentice-Hall. ISBN 0-13-914854-X

Cunninghis, R. N., & Best-Martini, E. (1996). *Quality assurance for activity programs* (2nd ed.). Ravensdale, WA: Idyll Arbor. ISBN 1-882883-23-3

Dattilo, J. (1999). *Leisure education program planning: A systematic approach* (2nd ed.). State College, PA: Venture Publishing. ISBN 1-892132-05-2

Dattilo, J. (2000). *Facilitation techniques in therapeutic recreation.* State College, PA: Venture Publishing. ISBN 1-892132-13-3

Dattilo, J. (2000). *Leisure education specific programs.* State College, PA: Venture Publishing. ISBN 1-892132-18-4

Dattilo, J. (2002). *Inclusive leisure services: Responding to the rights of people with disabilities.* State College, PA: Venture Publishing, Inc. ISBN 1-892132-27-3

Dattilo, J., & Murphy, W. D. (1987). *Behavior modification in therapeutic recreation.* State College, PA: Venture Publishing. ISBN 0-910251-21-5

Dehn, D. (1995). *Leisure step up.* Ravensdale, WA: Idyll Arbor. ISBN 1-882883-07-1

Edginton, C. R., Hudson, S., & Ford, P. M. (1999). *Leadership for recreation and leisure programs and settings* (2nd ed.). Champaign, IL: Sagamore Publishing. ISBN 1-57167-437-3

Elliot, J. E., & Elliott, J. A. (1999). *Recreation for older adults: Individual and group activities.* State College, PA: Venture Publishing. ISBN 1-892132-08-7

Epperson, A., Witt, A., & Hitzhusen, G. (Eds.). (1977). *Leisure counseling: An aspect of leisure education.* Springfield, IL: Charles C. Thomas Pub. ISBN 0-398-03619-5

Faulkner, R. W. (1991). *Therapeutic recreation protocol for treatment of substance addictions.* State College, VA: Venture Publishing. ISBN 0-910251-37-1.

Fine, A. H., & Fine, N. M. (1988). *Therapeutic recreation for exceptional children: Let me in, I want to play.* Springfield, IL: Charles C. Thomas Pub. ISBN 0-398-05479-7

Frye, V., & Peters, M. (1972). *Therapeutic recreation: Its theory, philosophy and practice.* Harrisburg, PA: Stackpole Books. ISBN 0-8117-1735-6

Grote, K., Hasl, M., Krider, R., & Mortensen, D. M. (1995). *Behavioral health protocols for recreational therapy.* Ravensdale, WA: Idyll Arbor. ISBN 1-882883-17-9

Haun, P. (1966). *Recreation: A medical viewpoint.* Arlington, VA: National Recreation and Parks Association. No ISBN.

Hawkins, B. A., May, M. E., & Rogers, N. B. (1996) *Therapeutic activity intervention with the elderly: Foundations and practices.* State College, PA: Venture Publishing. ISBN 0-910251-81-9

Hogberg, P., & Johnson, M. (1994). *Reference manual for writing rehabilitation therapy treatment plans.* State College, PA: Venture Publishing. ISBN 0-910251-67-3

Horvat, M., & Kalakian, L. (1996). *Assessment in adapted physical education and therapeutic recreation.* Dubuque, IA: Brown and Benchmark.

Howe-Murphy, R., & Charboneau, B. G. (1987). *Therapeutic recreation intervention: An ecological perspective.* Englewood Cliffs, NJ: Prentice-Hall. ISBN 0-13-914656-3

Hunt, V. V. (1955). *Recreation for the handicapped.* Englewood Cliffs, NJ: Prentice Hall. No ISBN.

Hutchinson, P., & Lord, J. (1979). *Recreation integration: Issues and alternatives in leisure services and community involvement.* Ontario, Canada: Leisurability Publication, Inc. ISBN 9-9690003-0-8

Kelland, J. (Ed.). (1995). *Protocols for recreation therapy.* State College, PA: Venture Publishing. ISBN 0-910251-73-8

Kelley, J. D. (Ed.). (1981). *Recreation programming for visually impaired children and youth.* New York: American Foundation for the Blind. ISBN 0-89128-106-1

Kennedy, D. W., Austin, D. R., & Smith, R. W. (2001). *Special recreation: Opportunities for people with disabilities* (4th ed.). Dubuque, IA: Wm C. Brown. ISBN 0-03-05456-1

Kloseck, M., & Crilly, R. G. (1997). *Leisure competence measure: Professional manual and users' guide.* London, Ontario: Leisure Competence Measure Data System. ISBN 0-9683306-0-6

Kraus, R., & Shank, J. (1992). *Therapeutic recreation service: Principles and practices* (4th ed.). Dubuque, IA: Wm. C. Brown, Publishers. ISBN 0-697-11026-5

Lawson, L. M., Coyle, C. P., & Ashton-Shaeffer, C. (2001). *Therapeutic recreation in special education: An IDEA for the future.* Alexandria, VA: American Therapeutic Recreation Association. ISBN 1-889435-16-3

Leitner, M. J., & Leitner, S. F. (1985). *Leisure in later life: A sourcebook for the provision of recreation services for elders.* New York: The Haworth Press. ISBN 0-86656-476-4

Loesch, L. C., & Wheeler, P. T. (1982). *Principles of leisure counseling.* Minneapolis, MN: Educational Media Corp. ISBN 0-932796-10-9

Malkin, M. J., & Howe, C. Z. (Eds.). (1993). *Research in therapeutic recreation: Concepts and methods.* State College, PA: Venture Publishing. ISBN 0-910251-53-3

Mascott, C. (2004). *The therapeutic recreation stress management primer.* State College, PA: Venture Publishing. ISBN 1-892132-44-3

McGuire, F. A., Boyd, R. K., & Tedrick, T. (2004) *Leisure and aging: Ulyssean living in later life* (3rd ed.). Champaign, IL: Sagamore Publishing. ISBN 1-57167-552-3

Melcher, S. (1999). *Introduction to writing goals and objectives.* State College, PA: Venture Publishing. ISBN 1-892132-10-9

Mobily, K. E., & MacNeil, R. D. (2002). *Therapeutic recreation and the nature of disabilities.* State College, PA: Venture Publishing. ISBN 1-892132-22-2

Navar, N., & Dunn, J. (Eds.). (1981). *Quality assurance: Concerns for therapeutic recreation.* Champaign, IL: Dept. of Leisure Studies, University of Illinois. No ISBN.

O'Dea-Evans, P. (1990). *Leisure education for addicted persons.* Algonquin, IL: Peapod Productions. No ISBN.

O'Morrow, J. S., & Carter, M. J. (1997). *Effective management in therapeutic recreation service.* State College, PA: Venture Publishing. ISBN 0-910251-87-8

O'Morrow, G. S., & Reynolds, R. P. (1989). *Therapeutic recreation: A helping profession* (3rd ed.). Englewood Cliffs, NJ: Prentice Hall. ISBN 0-13-914890-5

Rathbone, J. L., & Lucas, C. (1959). *Recreation in total rehabilitation.* Springfield, IL: Charles C. Thomas Publishing. ISBN 0-7216-5507-6

Reynolds, R. P., & O'Morrow, G. S. (1985). *Problems, issues and concerns in therapeutic recreation.* Englewood Cliffs, NJ: Prentice Hall, Inc. ISBN 0-13-717430-6

Riley, B. (Ed.). (1987). *Evaluation of therapeutic recreation through quality assurance.* State College, PA: Venture Publishing. ISBN 0-910251-18-5

Riley, B. (Ed.). (1991). *Quality management: Applications for therapeutic recreation.* State College, PA: Venture Publishing, Inc. ISBN 0-910251-47-9

Schleien, S. J., & Ray, M. T. (1988). *Community recreation and persons with disabilities: Strategies for integration.* Baltimore, MD: Paul Brookes Publishing. ISBN 0-933716-95-8

Schott, D., Burdett, J. D., Cook, B. J., Ford, K. S., & Orban, K. M. *Functional interdisciplinary—Transdisciplinary therapy (FITT) manual.* State College, PA: Venture Publishing. ISBN 1-892132-46-X

Shank, J., & Coyle, C. (2002). *Therapeutic recreation in health promotion and rehabilitation.* State College, PA: Venture Publishing. ISBN 0-697-11026-5

Smith, R. W., Austin, D. R., & Kennedy, D. W. (2001). *Inclusive and special recreation: Opportunities for persons with disabilities* (4th ed.). Boston, MA: McGraw Hill Publishing. ISBN 0-697-29495-1

Skalko, T. K., Mitchell, R. S., Kaye, A. G., & Dalton, M. J. (1994). *Basic guide to physical and psychiatric medications for recreational therapy.* Hattiesburg, MS: American Therapeutic Recreation Association. No ISBN.

Stein, T. A., & Sessoms, H. D. (1977). *Recreation for special populations* (2nd ed.). Boston: MA: Allyn and Bacon, Inc. ISBN 0-205-05690-3

Stumbo, N. J. (1997). *Leisure education III: More goal-oriented activities.* State College, PA: Venture Publishing, Inc. ISBN 0-9102251-91-6

Stumbo, N. J. (1998). *Leisure education IV: Activities for individuals with substance addictions.* State College, PA: Venture Publishing. ISBN 0-910251-93-2

Stumbo, N. J. (1999). *Intervention activities for at-risk youth.* State College, PA: Venture Publishing. ISBN 1-892132-07-9

Stumbo, N. J. (2001). *Professional issues in therapeutic recreation: On competence and outcomes.* Champaign, IL: Sagamore Publishing. ISBN: 1-57167-476-4

Stumbo, N. J. (2002). *Client assessment in therapeutic recreation services.* State College, PA: Venture Publishing. ISBN 1-892132-32-X

Stumbo, N. J. (2002). *Leisure education I: A manual of activities and resources* (2nd ed.). State College, PA: Venture Publishing. ISBN 1-8992132-25-7

Stumbo, N. J. (2002). *Leisure education II: More activities and resources* (2nd ed.). State College, PA: Venture Publishing. ISBN 1-892132-28-1

Stumbo, N. J. (Ed.). (2003). *Client outcomes in therapeutic recreation services.* State College, PA: Venture Publishing. ISBN 1-892132-43-5

Stumbo, N. J., & Peterson, C. A. (2004). *Therapeutic recreation program design: Principles and procedures* (4th ed.). San Francisco, CA: Benjamin Cummings. ISBN 0-8053-5497-2

Sylvester, C., Hemingway, J. L., Howe-Murphy, R., Mobily, K., & Shank, P. A. (1987). *Philosophy of therapeutic recreation: Ideas and issues.* Alexandria, VA: National Recreation and Park Association. No ISBN.

Sylvester, C., Voelkl, J. E., & Ellis, G. (2001). *Therapeutic recreation programming: Theory and practice.* State College, PA: Venture Publishing. ISBN 1-892132-20-6

Wehman, P. (Ed.). (1979). *Recreation programming for developmentally disabled persons.* Austin, TX: Pro-ed. ISBN 0-8391-1295-5

Wehman, P., & Schleien, S. (1981). *Leisure programs for handicapped persons: Adaptations, techniques and curriculum.* Austin, TX: Pro-ed. ISBN 0-8391-1643-8

Wilhite, B. C., & Keller, M. J. (2000). *Therapeutic recreation: Cases and exercises* (2nd ed.). State College, PA: Venture Publishing. ISBN 0-910251-50-9

Williams, B. (2004) *Assistive devices, adaptive strategies, and recreational activities for students with disabilities.* Champaign, IL: Sagamore Publishing. ISBN 1-57167-499-3

Winslow, R. M., & Halberg, K. L. (Eds.). (1992). *The management of therapeutic recreation services.* Arlington, VA: National Recreation and Parks Association. No ISBN.

Witt, P. A. (1979). *Community leisure services and disabled individuals.* Washington, DC: Hawkins & Associates, Inc. No ISBN.

Witt, P. A., & Ellis, G. D. (1989). *The leisure diagnostic battery: Users manual.* State College, PA: Venture Publishing. ISBN 0-910251-22-3

Wuerch, B. B., & Voeltz, L. M. (1982). *Longitudinal leisure skills for severely handicapped learners: The Ho'onanea curriculum component.* Baltimore, MD: University Park Press. ISBN 0-933716-26-5

Other Therapeutic Recreation Literature

American Therapeutic Recreation Association. (2000). *Standards for the practice of therapeutic recreation and self-assessment guide.* Alexandria, VA: Author. ISBN 1889435-02-3

American Therapeutic Recreation Association. (1990). *Code of ethics.* Alexandria, VA: Author.

National Council for Therapeutic Recreation Certification. (2004). *Candidate bulletin* [Electronic Version]. Thiells, New York: Author.

National Therapeutic Recreation Society. (1994). *Standards of practice for therapeutic recreation services.* Arlington, VA: National Recreation and Park Association.

National Therapeutic Recreation Society. (2003). *Standards of practice for therapeutic recreation services and annotated bibliography.* Arlington, VA: Author.

National Therapeutic Recreation Society. (1990). *Code of ethics and interpretive guidelines.* Arlington, VA: National Recreation and Park Association.

National Therapeutic Recreation Society. (1990). *Guidelines for the administration of therapeutic recreation services.* Arlington, VA: National Recreation and Park Association.

Therapeutic Recreation Journals and Periodicals

American Journal of Recreation Therapy. Weston, MA.

Annual in Therapeutic Recreation. American Therapeutic Recreation Association. Alexandria, VA.

Expanding Horizons in Therapeutic Recreation. University of Missouri Extension Division. Columbia, MO.

Therapeutic Recreation Journal. National Therapeutic Recreation Society/National Recreation and Park Association. Arlington, VA.

Recreation Literature

Allison, M. T., & Schneider, I. E. (Eds.). (2000). *Diversity and the recreation profession: Organizational perspectives.* State College, PA: Venture Publishing. ISBN 1-892132-14-1

Edginton, C. R., Hudson, S. D., & Ford, P. M. (1999). *Leadership in recreation and leisure service organizations* (2nd ed.). Champaign, IL: Sagamore Publishing. ISBN 1-57167-161-5

Edginton, C. R., Jordan, D. J., DeGraaf, D. G., & Edginton, S. R. (2002). *Leisure and life satisfaction: Foundational perspectives* (3rd ed.). Boston, MA: McGraw Hill. ISBN 0-07-235397-X

Godbey, G. (2003). *Leisure in your life: An exploration* (6th ed.). State College, PA: Venture Publishing. ISBN 1-892132-37-0

Iso-Ahola, S.E. (1980). *The social psychology of leisure and recreation.* Dubuque, IA: WM. C. Brown. ISBN 0-697-07167-7

Jordan, D. J. (2001). *Leadership in leisure services: Making a difference* (2nd ed.). State College, PA: Venture Publishing. ISBN 1-892132-21-4

Mannel, R. C., & Kleiber, D. (1997). *A social psychology of leisure.* State College, PA: Venture Publishing. ISBN 0-910251-88-6

Neulinger, J. (1974). *The psychology of leisure.* Springfield, IL: Charles C. Thomas. ISBN 0-398-03106-1

Russell, R. V. (2001) *Leadership in recreation* (2nd ed.). Boston, MA: McGraw Hill. ISBN 0-07-012330-6

Non-Therapeutic Recreation Literature

American Psychiatric Association. (2000). *Diagnostic and statistical manual of mental disorders* (4th ed. Text revision). Washington, DC: American Psychiatric Association. ISBN 0-89042-024-6

Blackman, J. A. (Ed.). (1983). *Medical aspects of developmental disabilities in children birth to three*. Iowa City, IA: Division of Developmental Disabilities, University of Iowa. No ISBN.

Davis, C. M. (1994). *Patient practitioner interaction: An experiential manual for developing the art of health care* (2nd ed.). Thorofare, NJ: Slack. ISBN 1-55642-232-6

Goldenson, R. M., Dunham, J. R., & Dunham, C. S. (Eds.). (1978). *Disability and rehabilitation handbook*. New York: MacGraw Hill. ISBN 0070236585

Grossman, H. J., & Tarjan, G. (Eds.). (1987). *AMA handbook on mental retardation*. Chicago, IL: American Medical Association. ISBN 0-89970-223-6

Johnson, D. W., & Johnson, F. (2002). *Joining together: Group therapy and group skills.* (8th ed.). Needham Heights, MA: Allyn & Bacon. ISBN 0205367402

Lewis, M. (1971). *Clinical aspects of child development*. Philadelphia, PA: Lea & Febiger. ISBN 0-8121-0313-0

National Center on Birth Defects and Developmental Disabilities. (2002) *Healthy people with disabilities: State information* [Brochure]. Atlanta, GA: Center for Disease Control and Prevention. No ISBN.

Mosey, A. C. (1973). *Activities therapy.* New York, NY: Raven Press. ISBN 0-911216-41-3

Paciorek, M. J., & Jones, J. A. (2001) *Disability sport & recreation resources* (3rd ed.). Traverse City, MI: Cooper Publishing. ISBN 1884125751

Scotch, R. K. (2001). *From goodwill to civil rights: Transforming federal disability policy* (2nd ed.). Philadelphia, PA: Temple University Press. ISBN 1-56639-896-7

Stolov, R., & Clowers, M. (1989). *Handbook of severe disability.* U.S. Department of Education Rehabilitation Services Administration, Government Printing Office Order #017-090-00054-2.

Tamparo, D. D., & Lewis, M. A. (2000). *Diseases of the human body* (3rd ed.). Philadelphia, PA: F. A. Davis Company. ISBN 0803605641

Vandara, D. R., & Egan, E. J. (Eds.). (1997). *Taber's cyclopdic medical dictionary* (18th ed.). Philadelphia, PA: F. A. Davis Company. ISBN 0-8036-813-8

SECTION TWO

Chapter Five
Warm-Up Items

This entire section provides you with almost 500 practice items. We have added 30% more items to the tests than are found in the second edition. This is to help you "overpractice," a method used in education to increase a person's competence (in this case at test-taking) and confidence level. We hope that it increases your ability to self-assess your strengths and weaknesses before taking the test, and, therefore, helps you to prepare in the most effective way possible.

However, we remind you once again, the items in this *Study Guide* represent the same basic format and content as the NCTRC exam, but this does not mean that they are the same items seen on the actual test. Our intent is to help you prepare, by giving you ample opportunity to test your own knowledge and skills before sitting for the test. Do not expect to see these exact items on the test.

Warm-Up Questions

The second section is divided into three chapters. The first chapter contains 90 warm-up items to get you started, especially if you have not taken a paper-and-pencil test for some time. The items come from all eight areas of the Content Outline, and are in no particular order. We advise that you complete the warm up in one sitting, practicing the test-taking strategies found in chapter three. This

section should take you about 30 minutes to complete. Notice the format of the items, as this will be the same format as on the actual NCTRC test. Complete the entire warm-up before looking at the answers. You will find the answers to the 90 items on page 90.

Practice Tests

The second chapter in this section has two sample practice tests of 90 items each. These practice sets are meant to be as close as possible to the NCTRC national test.

The NCTRC test will have 90 items in the following proportions:

Background	(8%)
Diagnostic Groupings and Populations Served	(15%)
Assessment	(15%)
Planning the Intervention	(15%)
Implementing the Individual Intervention Plan	(16%)
Documentation and Evaluation	(15%)
Organizing and Managing Services	(9%)
Advancement of the Profession	(7%)

Within the 90-item test, that means the number of items per area are:

Background	7
Diagnostic Groupings and Populations Served	13
Assessment	14
Planning the Intervention	14
Implementing the Individual Intervention Plan	14
Documentation and Evaluation	14
Organizing and Managing Services	8
Advancement of the Profession	6

We have designed this practice test in the same proportions as the actual NCTRC test. Our aim is to simulate the real test to the fullest extent possible. You may help this by completing the test in a quiet area, seated at a table or a desk, in one sitting. Again, this is a chance for you to try out the test-taking strategies in chapter three, and see which ones work for you.

This portion is meant to be completed in one sitting per practice test, and it will take approximately an hour each. (This is an estimate. The amount of time you take may be longer or shorter but should give you a good indication of how long the actual test will take you.)

After you have completed the two practice tests at 90 items each, you can score your own tests, with the answers located on page 91. Notice that the answers are grouped by the area of the Content Outline to which they are associated. Use these answer keys to help you diagnose your own strengths and weaknesses. Which knowledge area did you do well on? Which did you not? Does this correlate with what you know about your own level of knowledge? How many items, out of each practice test, did you miss?

Diagnostic and Remedial Items

You can use this information to move to the last chapter for more items. In chapter seven, there are 240 more items (30 questions per each of the eight areas). This time, items are grouped by the knowledge area under which they belong.

We did this quite purposely in case, say, you missed several items on Assessment in the practice tests but missed very few items about Documentation. You can use the Diagnostic and Review Test to take 30 more items on Assessment but not complete the Documentation section if you do not want to. Of course you can complete all the items, but our intent was to give you a bit more help in areas of potential weakness. Use this information to determine your weak areas that need more study and review.

Completing the cycle then, you can go back to chapter four on Basic Information to find more information and resources for your weak areas. Take time to understand what content is covered by the area, and find and use the resources suggested for gaining more knowledge. Make sure you leave enough time to access the materials and study in advance of the test.

Also make sure you read thoroughly the *Candidate's Bulletin* provided by the National Council for Therapeutic Recreation Certification to every test taker and found online at www.NCTRC.org. The *Candidate's Bulletin* explains all the details of the test administration and scoring, for example, how to register and when to expect score results. Write or call NCTRC directly for this and other information, as soon as you know when you will be taking the test. They are your best source of information about the certification examination, so always start there.

Warm-Up Items

The 90 sample questions that follow represent the types of questions included in the NCTRC Certification Exam. The purpose of this warm-up is to give you some indication of the topics that will be covered, as well as to provide some additional questions for practice purposes. These questions do not represent the *proportion* of actual test questions within each of the content categories, although it does contain the *same number of items* as does the NCTRC exam. You might considering timing yourself while taking this warm-up to see how long it takes you to answer 90 items.

Directions: For each question in this section, select the BEST answer of the choices given. Use the answer scoring sheet on pages 89-90 to record your answers. Use the answer scoring key on page 91 to check your answers after you have completed all of the items.

1. If a person believes that he/she does not have the right skills to complete a leisure experience, and then generalized this inadequacy to all other leisure behaviors, this person is exhibiting which of the following?

   (A) Leisure efficacy
   (B) Learned helplessness
   (C) Attributional leisure response
   (D) Extrinsic motivation

2. The medical term NPO is the abbreviation for

   (A) idiopathic diagnosis
   (B) nothing by mouth
   (C) normal parameters of oxygen
   (D) normal postoperative outpatient

3. According to the Leisure Ability model of service provision, the role of the therapeutic recreation specialist in leisure education can be as a(n)

   (A) leader, instructor, and therapist
   (B) instructor, advisor, and counselor
   (C) facilitator, advisor, and therapist
   (D) leader, facilitator, and counselor

4. What is likely to be the nature/role of a TRS in an acute care setting where the medical model is the mode of operation?

   (A) Design recreation participation programs for evening/weekend participation
   (B) Conduct one-on-one sessions with clients using leisure as a diversionary tool
   (C) Prepare individualized treatment programs based on physicians orders
   (D) Plan leisure education sessions so clients gain an awareness of leisure and life satisfaction

5. One of the major long-term effects of repeated use of inhalants is

    (A) extreme thirst
    (B) a strong reaction to sunlight
    (C) bruising of the forearms
    (D) improved sight acuity

6. Which statement describes the purpose of evidence-based practice?

    (A) Method of designing critical pathways
    (B) Process to control medical bills through reduction of services
    (C) Means of conducting near-patient research
    (D) Method to enhance client care through research application

Questions 7-9

The most widely accepted model for leisure education is composed of four components:

    I.   Leisure awareness
    II. Social interaction skills
    III. Leisure activity skills
    IV. Leisure resources

Refer to the component areas and choose the one(s) that best reflect the following goal statements.

7. To improve personal responsibility for leisure.

    (A) I
    (B) III
    (C) I, IV
    (D) III, IV

8. To improve community leisure skills

    (A) I
    (B) III
    (C) I, IV
    (D) III, IV

9. To gain an understanding of the effects of disability or illness on leisure behavior

    (A) I
    (B) III
    (C) I, IV
    (D) III, IV

10. Which of the following types of activity often is used in stress management programs?

   (A) Progressive muscle relaxation
   (B) Remotivation
   (C) Social skills training
   (D) Trust building

11. "Accessible" facilities become "usable" when the person with a disability can

   (A) expect to receive special treatment and services
   (B) function as independently as possible
   (C) socialize with individuals with similar disabilities
   (D) enter through the front door and use the restroom area

12. The three major characteristics of mental retardation are:

   (A) subaverage intellectual functioning, impairment in at least two adaptive skill areas, and evident before age 18
   (B) subaverage intellectual functioning, lack of physical coordination skills, and extraordinary facial features
   (C) subaverage social, intellectual, and physical functioning within community expectations
   (D) subaverage functioning in home, community, and school environments

13. The medical term "ad. lib." is the abbreviation for

   (A) as patient can tolerate
   (B) give freedom liberally
   (C) as often as possible
   (D) daily

14. A halfway house is used primarily for individuals who

   (A) need a balance of supervision and independence
   (B) are alcoholics
   (C) have mental retardation
   (D) have been diagnosed for at least two years

15. Which statement correctly identifies a criteria of an accessible parking space?

   (A) Accessible parking spaces are closest to the building entrance
   (B) Accessible parking may be distributed in a parking lot if greater access is achieved
   (C) Parking spaces and aisles are level with a slope no greater than 1:20
   (D) Parking spaces are at least 96 inches wide with adjacent access aisle of 68 inches

16. All of the following may be found in a therapeutic recreation department's policy and procedure manual, EXCEPT:

    (A) instructions for checking out and driving agency vehicles
    (B) treatment protocols for disability groups served by the department
    (C) guidelines for prescribing medications
    (D) information about staff recruiting, hiring, supervision, and firing

17. All of the following are ways to establish rapport with clients in an assessment interview, EXCEPT:

    (A) introduce yourself and explain your department
    (B) provide answers for the client
    (C) refer to the client by name
    (D) use body language that signals you are listening

18. An insurance carrier's cost control method of paying a prearranged amount for specific service, no matter what the actual cost of those services might be, is called

    (A) third-party reimbursement
    (B) prospective payment
    (C) cost allocation
    (D) unit cost

Questions 19-23

    I. Condition
    II. Behavior
    III. Criteria

   Written behavioral objectives that are measurable contain the three components listed above to specify what is expected from the patient/client. Examine each of the behavioral objectives below and determine whether a component is not measurable. If the behavioral objectives contains all three components, answer "D."

19. After the discussion group, the client will name three leisure resources in the local community, as judged by the CTRS.

    (A) I
    (B) II
    (C) III
    (D) It is written correctly.

20. The client will list several methods for improving time management.

    (A) I
    (B) III
    (C) I, III
    (D) It is written correctly.

21. While making a leisure activity collage, the client will name the necessary equipment.

    (A) I
    (B) II
    (C) III
    (D) It is written correctly.

22. When watering the plants, the client will use one cup of water once a week.

    (A) I
    (B) II
    (C) III
    (D) It is written correctly.

23. After losing a game, the patient will verbally congratulate the winner, 100% of the time.

    (A) I
    (B) II
    (C) III
    (D) It is written correctly.

24. The Americans with Disabilities Act of 1990 allows full and equal access by persons with disabilities to

    (A) any place of public accommodation, government, or private
    (B) state and federal buildings funded through public taxes
    (C) almost any public accommodation, but excludes recreation facilities
    (D) any recreation facility, whether public, private, or commercial

25. In a treatment protocol, the outcome criteria refers to

    (A) measurable changes brought about in a patient as a direct result of the intervention
    (B) how the assessment is conducted
    (C) the timing of the treatment evaluation
    (D) steps taken and services provided by the therapist to complete the protocol

26. The primary reason the American Therapeutic Recreation Association was created in 1984 was to

    (A) provide services to veterans returning from the Vietnam War
    (B) provide workshops and conferences for members to get CEUs
    (C) create the national certification examination for therapeutic recreation specialists
    (D) respond to concerns and issues of therapeutic recreation specialists working in clinical facilities

27. In 2001, the World Health Organization defined quality of life as:

    (A) return to health after a lengthy period of illness or disability
    (B) a person's perception of their overall health and well-being
    (C) the achievement of homeostatis
    (D) a major factor in ratings of patient satisfaction with health care services

28. Which type of facility has the highest bed occupancy rate of all long-term facilities?

    (A) Nursing homes
    (B) State facilities for individuals with developmental disabilities
    (C) Psychiatric hospitals
    (D) Physical medicine and rehabilitation centers

29. The director of the TR department conducted a study on the effectiveness of the previous marketing efforts done for therapeutic recreation services. The action taken by the director is called a marketing _____ .

    (A) audit
    (B) research schema
    (C) audience
    (D) tool

30. Individuals with mental retardation may have an unrealistic view of "self" because of which of the following?

    I.   They lack exposure to peer groups
    II. Their parents are often overprotective
    III. They have difficulty exploring and testing their own limits

    (A) I and II only
    (B) I and III only
    (C) II and III only
    (D) I, II, and III

31. The process of comparing the quantity of services provided with the amount of resources such as staff and time used is called

    (A) market segmenting
    (B) risk management
    (C) productivity measurement
    (D) analysis of care

32. Title II in the Americans with Disabilities Act of 1990 concerns discrimination in

    (A) recreation services and facilities
    (B) employment
    (C) education
    (D) transportation and communication services

Questions 33-34

Using the following categories of child development, choose the appropriate category in which the skill belongs.

     I.   Personal/social
    II. Adaptive/fine motor behavior
  III. Motor behavior
  IV. Language

33. Heeds his/her name

    (A) I
    (B) II
    (C) III
    (D) IV

34. Sits leaning forward on hands

    (A) I
    (B) II
    (C) III
    (D) IV

35. Which statement describes an intent or purpose common to both systems planning and quality improvement plans?

    (A) Each describes the relationship of the comprehensive program to individual treatment plans
    (B) Each outlines the relationship between the agency and departmental procedures
    (C) Both define the components of department programs
    (D) Each provides a systematic method of evaluative service delivery

36. The federal law that dictates currently the specifications for barrier free design is the

    (A) Architectural Barriers Act of 1968
    (B) Americans With Disabilities Act of 1990
    (C) Mandatory Inclusion Act of 1992
    (D) Barrier Free Environments Act of 2004

37. All of the following are examples of physical benefits of leisure participation EXCEPT:

    (A) Potential counteragent to negative lifestyle choices
    (B) Reduction of secondary disabilities
    (C) Improved health indicators such as bone density and joint mobility
    (D) Increase in high blood pressure and heart disease

38. What is the primary feature that distinguishes "therapeutic recreation" from "recreation?"

    (A) Setting in which interventions takes place
    (B) Purposeful nature of intervention to bring about behavioral change
    (C) Nature of the selected experiences to facilitate outcomes
    (D) Extent of time leaders prepare for interventions and follow-up after intervention

39. Which of the following is an example of clinical supervision?

    (A) Overseeing clients on a community out-trip
    (B) Overseeing clients during an in-house discussion group
    (C) Helping a junior professional become a better practitioner
    (D) Performing personnel evaluations on staff as least once per year

40. In 2001, the World Health Organization revamped its classification of human functioning and disablement. Called the International Classification of Functioning, Disability, and Health (ICF), it promotes

    (A) better medical care in third world countries
    (B) viewing human functioning and disablement from a biopyschosocial model of health
    (C) more active treatment for those with severe disabilities and terminal illnesses
    (D) therapeutic recreation as one of three services that promote quality of life

41. Which of the following client descriptions demonstrates the custodial or long-term care model of service delivery?

    (A) Individuals in acute psychiatric care
    (B) Day camp participants
    (C) Group home residents
    (D) Residents in a state mental health facility

42. The statement that identifies the agency's basic values and beliefs, and thus defines how it wants to be perceived by the public is called a

    (A) mission statement
    (B) scope of care statement
    (C) marketing statement
    (D) vision statement

43. Teenscope is a useful assessment to place adolescent clients into which types of therapeutic recreation programs?

    (A) Treatment
    (B) Social skills
    (C) Leisure resources
    (D) Leisure skills

44. The punishment model for corrections may adhere to the following motto:

    (A) "An eye for an eye"
    (B) "There is hope for everyone"
    (C) "A stitch in time saves nine"
    (D) "Do unto others as you would have them do unto you"

45. The *Comprehensive Accreditation Manual for Ambulatory Care,* the *Comprehensive Accreditation Manual for Behavioral Health Care,* and the *Comprehensive Accreditation Manual for Hospitals* are examples of standards manuals from which of the following organizations?

    (A) Agency for Healthcare Research and Quality (AHRQ)
    (B) Commission of Accreditation of Rehabilitation Facilities (CARF)
    (C) Joint Commission of Accreditation of Health Care Organizations (JCAHO)
    (D) Health Care Financing Administration (HCFA)

46. Unlike a municipal hospital, a private, for-profit hospital usually

    (A) specializes in one or a limited number of disorders
    (B) is operated by a governmental entity, such as a county
    (C) serves only children
    (D) serves individuals on a long-term basis

47. The Centers for Medicare and Medicaid Services (CMS) is the governmental agency responsible for

    (A) building collaborative initiatives between private and public hospitals
    (B) ensuring that patients within these programs pay their bills in a timely manner
    (C) reporting medical errors to the American Medical Association
    (D) regulatory review of hospitals that bill for Medicare and Medicaid recipients

48. The Americans with Disabilities Act includes provisions specifically regarding

    (A) employment, government services, and recreation
    (B) public transit, government services, and recreation
    (C) employment, government services, and public accommodations
    (D) employment, recreation, and public accommodations

49. Which act attempts to equalize mental health services with other medical services?

    (A) Mental Health Rehabilitation Act of 1996
    (B) Mental Health Parity Act of 1998
    (C) Mental Health Systems Act of 2001
    (D) Community Mental Health Systems Act of 2004

50. The Fox Activity Therapy Social Skills Baseline assessment was developed for use with which population?

    (A) Older individuals in nursing homes
    (B) Adults with developmental disabilities
    (C) Adults with mental health disturbances
    (D) Disabled children in inclusion programs

Questions 51-53

Using the following categories of child development, match the skill with the appropriate category.

    I.   personal/social
    II. adaptive/fine motor behavior
    III. motor behavior
    IV. language

51. Asks "why"

    (A) I only
    (B) II only
    (C) III only
    (D) IV only

52. Plays simple nursery games

    (A) I only
    (B) II only
    (C) III only
    (D) IV only

53. Walks with help

    (A) I only
    (B) II only
    (C) III only
    (D) IV only

54. Of the five major life areas (vocational, family, spiritual, social, leisure, and legal), leisure often is the _____ impacted by the use of substances.

    (A) last
    (B) second
    (C) first
    (D) third

55. The dividing vertebrae between being classified as a paraplegic and a quadriplegic is

    (A) C8, T1
    (B) T12, L1
    (C) T1, T2
    (D) T5, T6

56. Which of the following is NOT a possible means of transmission of HIV?

    (A) Donating blood
    (B) Unprotected sexual intercourse
    (C) Sharing drug injection paraphernalia
    (D) Mother to fetus

57. A disability that is present at birth is described as

    (A) congenital
    (B) adventitious
    (C) traumatic
    (D) acquired

58. One mistake in assessment many therapeutic recreation specialists make is to

    (A) improve the reliability of their assessment instrument
    (B) use the results of the assessment to place clients into programs
    (C) use an assessment that was intended for a different purpose
    (D) interview clients asking the questions in the same way every time

59. In assessment the most significant source of information is usually the

    (A) client
    (B) care giver
    (C) medical records
    (D) team members

60. Which of the following sets of standards was established by the field of therapeutic recreation to address the quality of service delivery?

    (A) Accreditation standards
    (B) Certification standards
    (C) Education standards
    (D) Standards of practice

61. Recreation participation programs are MOST appropriate for clients who need to

    (A) improve physical endurance
    (B) learn new leisure and recreation skills
    (C) practice social skills in an unstructured environment
    (D) become more aware of the role leisure plays in their lives

Questions 62-64

The most widely used leisure education model consists of the four major content areas. Select from the content areas listed below the one that BEST fits each of the following skills or knowledges.

    I. Leisure awareness
    II. Social interaction skills
    III. Leisure activity skills
    IV. Leisure resources

62. To demonstrate the ability to actively participate in a conversation for five minutes

    (A) I only
    (B) II only
    (C) III only
    (D) IV only

63. To demonstrate the ability to participate in a fitness activity of his/her choice

    (A) I only
    (B) II only
    (C) III only
    (D) IV only

64. To demonstrate the ability to use appropriate decision-making skills for leisure involvement

    (A) I only
    (B) II only
    (C) III only
    (D) IV only

65. While leading a reminiscing group at the long-term care facility, the TRS was unprepared to console/counsel a patient when he talked about a traumatic and difficult childhood. The TRS had inappropriately planned and analyzed the activity in which of the following domains?

    (A) Physical
    (B) Emotional
    (C) Social
    (D) Cognitive

66. Which of the following is an example of extinction that is meant to reduce a specific behavior?

    (A) Taking a client to the zoo when they are afraid of animals
    (B) Taking away a favorite toy when the client misbehaves
    (C) Talking to the client about antecedents, behaviors, and consequences
    (D) Applying the principle of negative reinforcement

Questions 67-68

    I. Condition
    II. Behavior
    III. Criteria

   Written behavioral objectives that are measurable contain the three components listed above to specify what is expected from the patient/client. Examine each of the behavioral objectives below and determine whether a component is not measurable. If the behavioral objective contains all three components, answer "D."

67. The client will verbally name three activities in which she will participate with a family member

    (A) I only
    (B) II only
    (C) III only
    (D) It is written correctly.

68. Upon completion of the program, the client will know one new leisure activity in which she would like to participate.

    (A) I only
    (B) II only
    (C) III only
    (D) It is written correctly.

69. Which statement identifies the primary factors considered as the number, length, and frequency of intervention sessions are planned?

    (A) The time constraints of the therapists and support staff
    (B) The number of clients served on the unit and space available
    (C) The case load and grand rounds of the physician on staff
    (D) The patients needs and nature of the program

70. In a team meeting in a physical rehabilitation unit, which therapist would most appropriately report that the client can perform activities of daily living (ADL) skills to a level suitable for discharge?

    (A) Physical therapist
    (B) Social worker
    (C) Therapeutic recreation specialist
    (D) Occupational therapist

71. A facility's master plan for treatment of each type of patient diagnosis is called a

    (A) protocol
    (B) critical pathway
    (C) written plan of operation
    (D) intervention

72. What is a primary outcome of completing a task analysis?

    (A) Behaviors needed to complete a skill are listed in a teaching sequence
    (B) A hierarchy of skills used in an activity are prepared
    (C) Each behavioral area exhibited in an activity is compared with one another
    (D) The time necessary for intervention is determined

73. Which set of standards governs the delivery of programs and services in the profession regardless of setting or population?

    (A) Critical pathways
    (B) Code of ethics
    (C) Plan of operations
    (D) Standards of practice

74. After the patient/client assessment has been completed, the next step in the programming process is to

    (A) write treatment summaries
    (B) analyze activities
    (C) identify the problem(s)
    (D) develop goals and objectives

Questions 75-77

During a discussion on the value of leisure, Albert said, "We need to change topics. I don't like this one. I think it's for sissies like the rest of you guys." Brandon said, " I feel like I'm benefiting from this discussion and I would like to continue." Cheryl said, "I'll go along with whatever the majority thinks."

75. Albert can be identified as displaying which of the following types of behavior?

    (A) Assertive
    (B) Non-assertive (passive)
    (C) Aggressive
    (D) Non-committal

76. Brandon can be identified as displaying which of the following types of behavior?

    (A) Assertive
    (B) Non-assertive (passive)
    (C) Aggressive
    (D) Non-committal

77. Cheryl can be identified as displaying which of the following types of behavior?

    (A) Assertive
    (B) Non-assertive (passive)
    (C) Aggressive
    (D) Non-committal

Questions 78-81

    I. Assessment of problem area
    II. Task analysis of behavior necessary to achieve skills
    III. Introduction to and rationale of learning the skills
    IV. Demonstration and modeling of specific social behaviors
    V. Practice and rehearsal of new behavior
    VI. Provision of feedback and reinforcement of behavior
    VII. Generalization of skill to variety of situations

Use the teaching sequence above for Social Skills Training to answer the questions or statement below.

78. In this step, the TRS lists, in sequential order, the actions required to perform the social skill.

    (A) I only
    (B) II only
    (C) I, II, and III only
    (D) V, VI, and VII only

79. In this step, the TRS reviews and corrects inappropriate actions taken by the clients.

    (A) I only
    (B) V only
    (C) VI only
    (D) VII only

80. In this step, the TRS may discuss with clients ways they can use these behaviors in community settings after discharge.

    (A) I, II and III only
    (B) V and VI only
    (C) VI only
    (D) VII only

81. In this step, the TRS talks about the need for social skills in most leisure environments.

    (A) I only
    (B) III only
    (C) III and VI only
    (D) VII only

82. The TRS is working with a group of chemically dependent teenagers. The goal of the program is "To gain an understanding of the importance of leisure." The TRS decides to use an activity called "Twenty Things I Love To Do." This is an example of

    (A) reality therapy
    (B) assertiveness
    (C) values clarification
    (D) bibliotherapy

83. During a planning session for a community outing, the TRS told the group that each person was a team member and was responsible for making decisions and helping to plan the outing. The TRS was using which of the following types of leadership style?

    (A) Autocratic
    (B) Democratic
    (C) Laissez-faire
    (D) Motivational

84. When using behavior modification with an emotionally disturbed female child, the TRS teaches her how to successfully interact with male peers after she has learned how to successfully interact with female peers. What behavior modification technique is the TRS using?

    (A) Shaping
    (B) Modeling
    (C) Extinction
    (D) Chaining

85. The TRS asked clients who had recently experienced strokes to identify their highest priorities, set goals, and develop an action plan for their leisure. The technique this TRS was teaching is called

    (A) goal orientation
    (B) self-actualization
    (C) time management
    (D) remotivation

86. Observation of overt behavior and the learning of new behavior is a focus of _____ theory.

    (A) psychoanalytic
    (B) cognitive-behavioral
    (C) behavioristic
    (D) growth

87. Leisure is often a social experience. Which of the following is a benefit usually received from friendships or social support networks?

    (A) Greater sense of well-being
    (B) Earlier onset of disease
    (C) Maximizing the impact of stress on health
    (D) Reduction of rewards received from leisure experiences

88. Debriefing a therapeutic recreation activity or session is important because it allows clients time to

    (A) socialize with peers so the specialist can make additional systematic observations
    (B) analyze the intent of the activity and draw conclusions about their own behavior
    (C) think about the purpose of the activity and how it relates to their past
    (D) take control of the activity and decide what rules and regulations will be followed

89. People who are intrinsically motivated in their leisure tend to

    (A) avoid situations in which they are challenged to demonstrate a certain skill level
    (B) seek challenges equal to their competence
    (C) avoid situations which may result in negative feedback about their performance
    (D) seek situations that are easily accomplished or quickly won

90. A therapeutic recreation specialist may increase the client's sense of control in all of the following ways EXCEPT

    (A) asking what type of community event the person would like to attend
    (B) giving the client an important role in planning to attend the event
    (C) asking the client to take part in the meal preparation
    (D) placing the sign-up sheet in the main activity room so all can find it

Warm-Up Items
Answer Scoring Sheet

1. Ⓐ Ⓑ Ⓒ Ⓓ   14. Ⓐ Ⓑ Ⓒ Ⓓ   27. Ⓐ Ⓑ Ⓒ Ⓓ   40. Ⓐ Ⓑ Ⓒ Ⓓ

2. Ⓐ Ⓑ Ⓒ Ⓓ   15. Ⓐ Ⓑ Ⓒ Ⓓ   28. Ⓐ Ⓑ Ⓒ Ⓓ   41. Ⓐ Ⓑ Ⓒ Ⓓ

3. Ⓐ Ⓑ Ⓒ Ⓓ   16. Ⓐ Ⓑ Ⓒ Ⓓ   29. Ⓐ Ⓑ Ⓒ Ⓓ   42. Ⓐ Ⓑ Ⓒ Ⓓ

4. Ⓐ Ⓑ Ⓒ Ⓓ   17. Ⓐ Ⓑ Ⓒ Ⓓ   30. Ⓐ Ⓑ Ⓒ Ⓓ   43. Ⓐ Ⓑ Ⓒ Ⓓ

5. Ⓐ Ⓑ Ⓒ Ⓓ   18. Ⓐ Ⓑ Ⓒ Ⓓ   31. Ⓐ Ⓑ Ⓒ Ⓓ   44. Ⓐ Ⓑ Ⓒ Ⓓ

6. Ⓐ Ⓑ Ⓒ Ⓓ   19. Ⓐ Ⓑ Ⓒ Ⓓ   32. Ⓐ Ⓑ Ⓒ Ⓓ   45. Ⓐ Ⓑ Ⓒ Ⓓ

7. Ⓐ Ⓑ Ⓒ Ⓓ   20. Ⓐ Ⓑ Ⓒ Ⓓ   33. Ⓐ Ⓑ Ⓒ Ⓓ   46. Ⓐ Ⓑ Ⓒ Ⓓ

8. Ⓐ Ⓑ Ⓒ Ⓓ   21. Ⓐ Ⓑ Ⓒ Ⓓ   34. Ⓐ Ⓑ Ⓒ Ⓓ   47. Ⓐ Ⓑ Ⓒ Ⓓ

9. Ⓐ Ⓑ Ⓒ Ⓓ   22. Ⓐ Ⓑ Ⓒ Ⓓ   35. Ⓐ Ⓑ Ⓒ Ⓓ   48. Ⓐ Ⓑ Ⓒ Ⓓ

10. Ⓐ Ⓑ Ⓒ Ⓓ   23. Ⓐ Ⓑ Ⓒ Ⓓ   36. Ⓐ Ⓑ Ⓒ Ⓓ   49. Ⓐ Ⓑ Ⓒ Ⓓ

11. Ⓐ Ⓑ Ⓒ Ⓓ   24. Ⓐ Ⓑ Ⓒ Ⓓ   37. Ⓐ Ⓑ Ⓒ Ⓓ   50. Ⓐ Ⓑ Ⓒ Ⓓ

12. Ⓐ Ⓑ Ⓒ Ⓓ   25. Ⓐ Ⓑ Ⓒ Ⓓ   38. Ⓐ Ⓑ Ⓒ Ⓓ   51. Ⓐ Ⓑ Ⓒ Ⓓ

13. Ⓐ Ⓑ Ⓒ Ⓓ   26. Ⓐ Ⓑ Ⓒ Ⓓ   39. Ⓐ Ⓑ Ⓒ Ⓓ   52. Ⓐ Ⓑ Ⓒ Ⓓ

Warm-Up Items
Answer Scoring Sheet

53. Ⓐ Ⓑ Ⓒ Ⓓ   66. Ⓐ Ⓑ Ⓒ Ⓓ   79. Ⓐ Ⓑ Ⓒ Ⓓ

54. Ⓐ Ⓑ Ⓒ Ⓓ   67. Ⓐ Ⓑ Ⓒ Ⓓ   80. Ⓐ Ⓑ Ⓒ Ⓓ

55. Ⓐ Ⓑ Ⓒ Ⓓ   68. Ⓐ Ⓑ Ⓒ Ⓓ   81. Ⓐ Ⓑ Ⓒ Ⓓ

56. Ⓐ Ⓑ Ⓒ Ⓓ   69. Ⓐ Ⓑ Ⓒ Ⓓ   82. Ⓐ Ⓑ Ⓒ Ⓓ

57. Ⓐ Ⓑ Ⓒ Ⓓ   70. Ⓐ Ⓑ Ⓒ Ⓓ   83. Ⓐ Ⓑ Ⓒ Ⓓ

58. Ⓐ Ⓑ Ⓒ Ⓓ   71. Ⓐ Ⓑ Ⓒ Ⓓ   84. Ⓐ Ⓑ Ⓒ Ⓓ

59. Ⓐ Ⓑ Ⓒ Ⓓ   72. Ⓐ Ⓑ Ⓒ Ⓓ   85. Ⓐ Ⓑ Ⓒ Ⓓ

60. Ⓐ Ⓑ Ⓒ Ⓓ   73. Ⓐ Ⓑ Ⓒ Ⓓ   86. Ⓐ Ⓑ Ⓒ Ⓓ

61. Ⓐ Ⓑ Ⓒ Ⓓ   74. Ⓐ Ⓑ Ⓒ Ⓓ   87. Ⓐ Ⓑ Ⓒ Ⓓ

62. Ⓐ Ⓑ Ⓒ Ⓓ   75. Ⓐ Ⓑ Ⓒ Ⓓ   88. Ⓐ Ⓑ Ⓒ Ⓓ

63. Ⓐ Ⓑ Ⓒ Ⓓ   76. Ⓐ Ⓑ Ⓒ Ⓓ   89. Ⓐ Ⓑ Ⓒ Ⓓ

64. Ⓐ Ⓑ Ⓒ Ⓓ   77. Ⓐ Ⓑ Ⓒ Ⓓ   90. Ⓐ Ⓑ Ⓒ Ⓓ

65. Ⓐ Ⓑ Ⓒ Ⓓ   78. Ⓐ Ⓑ Ⓒ Ⓓ

Warm-Up Items
Answer Scoring Key

1. **B**	14. **A**	27. **B**	40. **B**	53. **C**	66. **B**	79. **C**
2. **B**	15. **B**	28. **C**	41. **D**	54. **C**	67. **A**	80. **D**
3. **B**	16. **C**	29. **A**	42. **A**	55. **C**	68. **B**	81. **B**
4. **C**	17. **B**	30. **D**	43. **D**	56. **A**	69. **D**	82. **C**
5. **A**	18. **B**	31. **C**	44. **A**	57. **A**	70. **D**	83. **B**
6. **D**	19. **D**	32. **D**	45. **C**	58. **C**	71. **B**	84. **D**
7. **A**	20. **C**	33. **D**	46. **A**	59. **A**	72. **A**	85. **C**
8. **D**	21. **C**	34. **C**	47. **D**	60. **D**	73. **D**	86. **C**
9. **A**	22. **D**	35. **D**	48. **C**	61. **C**	74. **C**	87. **A**
10. **A**	23. **D**	36. **B**	49. **B**	62. **B**	75. **C**	88. **B**
11. **B**	24. **A**	37. **D**	50. **B**	63. **C**	76. **A**	89. **B**
12. **A**	25. **A**	38. **B**	51. **D**	64. **A**	77. **B**	90. **D**
13. **A**	26. **D**	39. **C**	52. **A**	65. **B**	78. **B**	

Chapter Six
Practice Tests

This chapter contains two practice tests of 90 items each, similar to what you will experience with the NCTRC test. In the introduction to the second section, we listed the proportions that each area will be represented with items. We have followed those proportions in developing the following practice tests.

Our intent of these practice tests is to simulate how taking the test will feel. We suggest you take each practice test in one sitting, so you will become aware of your own reactions to sitting and concentrating for this period of time.

Find a quiet space that you can occupy for a period of about an hour and a half and take the first practice test. Use the guidelines in chapter three to make efficient and effective use of your time. Use the scoring sheet on page 110 to mark your answers. When you are finished with the first practice test, you can find the answers on page 112.

You will note, as you score your first practice test, that the scoring key is arranged in such a fashion as to help you determine in which area(s) you may need more work. You will be able to determine quite quickly in which area(s) you have done well and in which area(s) you have not done well.

Then use the same pattern to take the second practice test. Take the test, which starts on page 114. Then score your test using the scoring key on page 130.

After both practice tests are completed, compare your answers on the scoring keys. Are there one or more areas that you did really well? Are there one or more areas in which you need additional study? These scoring keys are meant to be used as diagnostic tools to help you determine your strong and weak areas (as indicated by the items on the practice tests). Do remember that you will NOT see these same items on the actual NCTRC exam.

Once you have determined your strong and weak areas, you can use the Diagnostic and Review questions found in chapter seven.

In chapter seven, there are 30 questions per each of the eight knowledge areas. Use these to help you determine if you do, in fact, need more preparation before taking the actual NCTRC exam. If you find you need more information about a specific area, return to chapter four, reread the information, and refer to the listing of resources given for each area. You may find that obtaining and reviewing a copy of these resources will be beneficial to you. Leave enough time to become familiar with these areas before you take the actual NCTRC test.

After additional study, you may want to retake the practice test or diagnostic items to see if you score better than the first time you tried. Try not to focus on these exact questions, but on the content which they represent. Always strive for a thorough understanding of the content, not just a quick memorization of the facts.

Practice Test 1

The sample questions that follow represent the types of questions included in the NCTRC Certification Exam. The purpose of this Practice Test is to give you some indication of what it will feel to take the actual NCTRC exam. The length of the test, and content and format of the questions is close to that of the national test.

Directions: For each question in this section, select the best of the answer choices given. Use the answer sheet on page 110 to record your answers. Use the scoring key on page 112 to score your answers.

1. If a person believes that he/she does not have adequate skills to play softball, and then generalizes this inadequacy to all physical activity, this person is exhibiting which of the following?

   (A) Leisure efficacy
   (B) Learned helplessness
   (C) Attributional leisure response
   (D) Intrinsic motivation

2. Reality orientation is a technique used to combat what symptom(s)?

   (A) Delusions
   (B) Irresponsibility and immaturity
   (C) Chronic fatigue and stress
   (D) Confusion

3. Diagnostic or treatment protocols, when properly researched and supported, have the potential to _____ therapeutic recreation practice.

   (A) assess
   (B) standardize
   (C) evaluate
   (D) counteract

4. A _____ is a document kept within a client's medical record that specifies the actions to be taken on the behalf of and by the client in order to reach his/her goals.

   (A) critical pathway
   (B) written plan of operation
   (C) protocol
   (D) treatment plan

5. Which of the following organizations allows for chapter affiliation by local groups of TRSs?

   (A) National Therapeutic Recreation Society (NTRS)
   (B) American Therapeutic Recreation Association (ATRA)
   (C) Recreation Therapy Section (RTS)
   (D) National Council for Therapeutic Recreation Certification (NCTRC)

6.   If a client assessment produces results that are reliable, it means that

(A) the content of the assessment matches the content of the intervention program
(B) the same client will receive about the same score if given the assessment twice
(C) clients are placed into the most appropriate programs to meet their needs
(D) two different assessments will produce the same results over time

Question 7

Sample discharge summary:

Pt. was referred to TR program due to lack of appropriate social skills at peer level and complaints of boredom. Pt. participated in Social Skills Training programs on a weekly basis and Leisure Opportunities programs on a daily basis for a duration of five weeks. Pt. is enrolled in two community-based leisure programs. TRS will follow-up in three weeks to monitor client progress in community.

7.   Which one of the following components is missing from the discharge summary?

(A) Major client goals or problems
(B) Services received by the client
(C) Client attainment of goals
(D) Plans for post-discharge involvement

8.   Alcoholism is characterized by

(A) physical dependence on alcohol and interruption in typical life functions
(B) drinking 3-7 drinks per day
(C) spending more than 20% of income on alcoholic beverages
(D) repeated intoxication in public

9.   A TRS may use which of the following resources to determine a client's leisure interests?

I.   Administration of an activity interest inventory to a client
II.   Interviews with the client regarding leisure interests
III. Interviews with the client's family or significant others

(A) I and II only
(B) I and III only
(C) II and III only
(D) I, II and III

10.   When assessing a child's ability to remain seated during a 30-minute activity, the TRS would look for which of the following behavioral characteristics?

(A) Duration of behavior
(B) Frequency of behavior
(C) Intensity of behavior
(D) Rate of the behavior

Questions 11-12

The most widely used therapeutic recreation service model consists of the three areas of service provision listed below. Select the one that BEST fits each of the following goal statements.

   I.   Functional intervention
  II.   Leisure education
 III.   Recreation participation

11.   To provide leisure opportunities that allows the client freedom to voluntarily participate

   (A)   I only
   (B)   II only
   (C)   III only
   (D)   I and II only

12.   To increase ability to refrain from hitting others

   (A)   I only
   (B)   II only
   (C)   III only
   (D)   I and II only

13.   What is the relationship between quality of life, functional domains, and client health status?

   (A)   The relationship is determined by service provided
   (B)   The quality of life is determined by intervention selected to achieve client goals
   (C)   The relationship is determined by the therapist's ability to properly assess client needs
   (D)   The quality of life is enhanced when clients experience improved abilities that promote healthy behaviors

14.   The *Diagnostic and Statistical Manual of Mental Disorders IVTR* classifies which type of disorders?

   (A)   Mental illness
   (B)   Mental retardation
   (C)   Cognitive impairments
   (D)   Learning disabilities

15.   Which of the following are true statements about implementing therapeutic recreation programs for clients?

   I.   The specialist should know several different facilitation techniques in order to select the most appropriate one for a particular group.
  II.   The facilitation technique selected by the specialist depends upon the abilities, limitations and needs of the clients.
 III.   Each client will vary in the amount he/she may benefit from a particular type of facilitation technique.

IV. Facilitation techniques have been developed in order to provide the most beneficial therapeutic activities.

(A) I only
(B) II only
(C) I, II, III only
(D) I, II, III and IV

16. A person who had a(n) _____ disorder may have limited, inflexible behaviors that inhibit his/her ability to interact with others and deal with certain aspects of his/her environment.

(A) Circulatory
(B) Attention deficit
(C) Nervous
(D) Orthopedic

17. The Leisure Competence Measure (LCM) parallels the format of which of the following client assessments?

(A) Functional Independence Measure (FIM)
(B) Rancho Los Amigos Scale
(C) Brief Leisure Rating Scale (BLRS)
(D) Leisure Barriers Inventory (LBI)

18. The basic principles of Remotivation as a therapy include which of the following?

  I. Warm, caring, concerned environment
 II. Confrontation with other members of peer group
III. Personal recollections of the topic of the day
 IV. Connections between past and present reality

(A) I only
(B) II only
(C) I, III and IV only
(D) I, II, III, and IV

19. A TRS should observe which of the following procedures when transferring an individual with a physical disability?

  I. Asking how and what type of assistance is needed
 II. Maintaining a firm grasp on the individual throughout all points of the transfer
III. Keeping the majority of the individual's weight as close as possible to the TRS's own body

(A) I and II only
(B) I and III only
(C) II and III only
(D) I, II and III

20. Older adults often need an extended rest period following physical exertion because they

    (A) are less motivated to continue to exercise
    (B) require longer to return to a state of homeostasis after an activity
    (C) fail to properly warm up prior to the exercise
    (D) tend to overexert during physical activities

21. Which of the following assessments was designed to coincide with the Functional Independence Measure (FIM)?

    (A) Leisure Diagnostic Battery (LDB)
    (B) Comprehensive Evaluation in Recreational Therapy Scale (CERT)
    (C) Leisure Competence Measure (LCM)
    (D) Leisure Activities Blank (LAB)

22. In a psychiatric short-term unit, during a team meeting it is reported, "The patient is responding to medication and is stable for referral to day treatment." Who would MOST LIKELY make this statement during the staffing?

    (A) Physiatrist
    (B) Psychiatrist
    (C) Psychiatric social worker
    (D) Psychiatric nurse

23. The TRS has developed protocols for each diagnostic category of clients served on the unit. Which statement best describes how the TRS would use the protocols in designing individual treatment plans?

    (A) The team would determine the length of time of each modality on a critical pathway
    (B) The therapist would select assessment/evaluation tools to measure protocol outcome
    (C) The therapist would use the protocol to assist in the selection of activity content and process
    (D) The protocol would be used by the team to evaluate the individualized treatment plan

24. Which of the following is NOT a result of chronic stress?

    (A) Adrenal glands secrete corticoids that inhibit digestion
    (B) Cellular tissue repair is made more quickly
    (C) Reproduction system is impaired
    (D) Immune system is weakened

25. A TRS wants to assess a patient's/client's ability to follow simple directions. The TRS should assess behavior from which of the following domains?

    (A) Cognitive
    (B) Physical
    (C) Emotional
    (D) Social

26. The specialist leads a group of clients in a form of stress management that has them tense certain muscles for five to seven seconds, then relax. What is this type of stress management called?

    (A) Progressive relaxation
    (B) Yoga
    (C) Meditation
    (D) Sensory stimulation

27. According to the Americans with Disabilities Act, if a child with a disability needs assistance to participate in a day camp program which the TRS offers, the TRS must provide the following, depending on the child's needs:

    I.   Someone to assist the child in program participation
    II. Someone to assist the child in toileting
    III. Someone to assist the child in feeding
    IV. Adapted equipment if the TRS is providing equipment for other participants

    (A) I only
    (B) I and II only
    (C) I, II, and III only
    (D) I and IV only

28. The head of the therapeutic recreation department in a center that serves older adults who come for services during the day and go to their own home at night would use which of the following manuals to assure compliance with external accreditation standards?

    (A) *Behavioral Health Standards* (CARF)
    (B) *Adult Day Services Manual* (CARF)
    (C) *Comprehensive Accreditation Manual for Long-Term Care* (JCAHO)
    (D) *Accreditation Manual for Assisted Living* (JCAHO)

29. Which of the following documents should be evaluated and updated on a regular basis?

    I.   Job announcement
    II. Performance appraisal
    III. Job description

    (A) I only
    (B) II only
    (C) II and III only
    (D) I, II, and III

30. The symptoms of anorexia nervosa are

    (A) refusal to eat, loss of hair, frequent vomiting
    (B) binge eating, depression, weighing constantly
    (C) secretive behavior, hyperactivity, depression
    (D) loss of 25 percent body weight, growth of fine body hair

31. A TRS in a correctional institution may emphasize programming based on improving the individual's self-efficacy in coping with high-risk situations that may trigger reincarceration. An example of a program title suited for this purpose is

(A) Relapse Prevention Strategies
(B) Total Body Workout
(C) Competitive Volleyball
(D) Bibliotherapy

32. Which of the following best represents the Activity Therapy model of therapeutic recreation service delivery?

(A) The focus of programs is on activity skills acquisition.
(B) Similar disciplines, such as art, music, dance and recreation therapy, are housed in one department.
(C) The philosophy is "All recreation is therapeutic."
(D) The focus of programs is on improving the functional independence of clients.

33. The discrepancy between the mental age (MA) and the chronological age (CA) for persons with mental retardation

(A) becomes less noticeable with age
(B) becomes more noticeable with age
(C) influences the quality of the materials used in recreation equipment
(D) determines the facility to be used

34. All programs in therapeutic recreation should be based on

(A) resources
(B) client need
(C) client interests
(D) clinician skill

Questions 35-36

Using the Axis descriptions used in the *DSM IV*, on which Axis will the following information be reported?

    I.   Axis I—Clinical Disorders
    II. Axis II—Personality Disorders; Mental Retardation
    III. Axis III—General Medical Conditions
    IV. Axis IV—Psychosocial and Environmental Problems

35. Substance-related disorders

(A) Axis I
(B) Axis II
(C) Axis III
(D) Axis IV

36. Post-partum depression

    (A) Axis I
    (B) Axis II
    (C) Axis III
    (D) Axis IV

37. A person who had a brain injury and now has problems speaking is considered to have

    (A) autism
    (B) an aneurysm
    (C) aphasia
    (D) an occlusion

38. All of the following would be principles of effective time management, EXCEPT:

    (A) minimize time wasters
    (B) procrastinate at least once a day
    (C) create an ongoing list of goals and priorities
    (D) keep an organizer or calendar close at hand

39. One of the basic principles of assertiveness training is

    (A) if allowed, people will tend to be aggressive toward one another
    (B) that the majority of people need a significant amount of training in social skills
    (C) that each individual should be able to stand up for his/her rights, while acknowledging those of others
    (D) that most stress is experienced when trying to work with others

40. When choosing an assessment instrument, the TRS first needs to determine the instrument's

    (A) reliability
    (B) validity
    (C) stability
    (D) purpose

41. The TRS had eight four-year-old children who had behavioral problems (like kicking, biting, and spitting on others) compete with each other on two bowling teams. Instead of realizing the children had difficulty interacting in the _____ interaction pattern and having them practice skills at that level, she had them participating in an activity that required a _____ interaction pattern, and thus, the children got aggressive and the activity failed.

    (A) Aggregate, intergroup
    (B) Intraindividual, extraindividual
    (C) Aggregate, interindividual
    (D) Cooperative, competitive

Question 42

Use the following statement to answer item 42.

    I.   Analyze the activity as it is normally engaged in.
    II. When completing an activity analysis, rate the activity as compared to all other activities.
    III. Analyze the activity, first, without regard for any specific disability group per se.
    IV. Analyze the activity with regard to the minimal level of skills required for basic, successful participation.

42. Which of the following statements represent principles of activity analysis?

    (A) I, II, III, and IV
    (B) I, II, and III only
    (C) I and II only
    (D) II, III, and IV only

43. After administering the Leisure Diagnostic Battery (LDB), the TRS scored the client's subscales and found that the client had an external locus of control, among other findings. Which of the following client statements would confirm these assessment results?

    (A) "I am a very goal-oriented person."
    (B) "I want you to make that decision for me."
    (C) "I am saving money to go on a vacation next month."
    (D) "I followed up on our conversation and I'm entering that writing contest next week."

44. The Minimum Data Set (MDS) assessment is required by which of the following agencies?

    (A) Joint Commission on Accreditation of Healthcare Organizations (JCAHO)
    (B) Rehabilitation Accreditation Commission (CARF)
    (C) Centers for Medicare and Medicaid Services (CMS)
    (D) National Therapeutic Recreation Society (NTRS)

45. A treatment plan should be entered into the medical chart after

    (A) seeing the patient once
    (B) conferring with the physician
    (C) the patient/legal guardian has agreed to the treatment plan
    (D) the patient has been in the hospital for a week

46. Which of the following are typical parts of a diagnostic protocol?

    (A) Assessment, planning, implementation, evaluation
    (B) Subjective, objective, analysis, planning
    (C) Comprehensive program descriptions and specific program descriptions
    (D) Client problems, assessment criteria, process criteria, and outcomes criteria

47. Utilization review in hospitals is the process of

    (A) recruiting, interviewing and hiring new specialists from various disciplines
    (B) changing from retrospective payments to managed care
    (C) evaluating the most efficient and effective use of resources
    (D) making sure all professionals attend professional conferences in their discipline

Question 48

Consider the following four categories of assessment:

    I. Leisure Attitudes and Barriers
    II. Functional Abilities
    III. Leisure Activity Skills
    IV. Leisure Interests and Participation Patterns

48. Which of the following categories would be most appropriate for a therapeutic recreation program that includes treatment/prescriptive programs, lifetime recreation skills, and leisure values programs?

    (A) I only
    (B) II and III only
    (C) I, II, and III only
    (D) I, II, III, and IV

49. The process by which a nongovernmental agency or association grants recognition to an individual who has met certain predetermined qualifications specified by that agency or association is called _____ .

    (A) licensure
    (B) accreditation
    (C) certification
    (D) registration

50. Which of the following assessments would be located in the category of Leisure Interests and Participation Patterns?

    (A) General Recreation Screening Tool (GRST)
    (B) Leisure Satisfaction Scale (LSS)
    (C) Brief Leisure Rating Scale (BLRS)
    (D) State Technical Institute Leisure Assessment Process (STILAP)

51. One reason that client assessment is important to therapeutic recreation service delivery is it

    (A) empowers clients to prepare for life changes
    (B) relates directly to program evaluation
    (C) helps clients achieve their goals by being placed in the most appropriate programs
    (D) analyzes which programs are best for certain groups of clients

52. The TRS observes the client's ability to complete a five-minute walking endurance test. What functional behavior is being assessed?

   (A) Cognitive
   (B) Physical
   (C) Social
   (D) Emotional

53. Which statement best describes an outcome of completing activity analysis?

   (A) Activities are referenced according to their difficulty
   (B) The amount of time necessary for the client to acquire the skill is determined
   (C) The skills necessary to perform the activity are identified
   (D) The types of adaptations needed by clients are determined

54. For which group of clients is recreation participation programs most suited?

   (A) Clients who need to improve physical well-being and health
   (B) Clients who need to develop new leisure time skills
   (C) Clients who need to develop comfort in social settings
   (D) Clients who need to practice interaction skills in unstructured situations

55. In the process of developing an assessment instrument, the TRS observes and rates the client. Then the first TRS has another TRS observe and rate the client on the same functional behaviors. The ratings are then compared, with a nearly perfect coefficient. What instrument characteristic is being determined?

   (A) Validity
   (B) Reliability
   (C) Usability
   (D) Practicality

56. Which of the following is a formative program evaluation question?

   (A) What unanticipated events or outcomes occurred in this program that were not part of the program plan?
   (B) Did the sequence of activities appear to be logical and appropriate?
   (C) How much time will be allotted for the program next time it is offered?
   (D) Are there enough resources for the remainder of the program?

57. Evaluation is conducted on specific individual programs in order to

   (A) provide systematic information for future program decisions
   (B) provide systematic information on client regression
   (C) increase validity and reliability of client assessment procedures
   (D) develop individual client treatment plans

58. The TRS was offered free tickets for patients/clients to attend a special performance of a play during the afternoon, but instead chose to have the patients/clients pay and attend a night performance. The TRS was demonstrating which of the following mainstreaming principles?

    (A) Integration
    (B) Normalization
    (C) Least restrictive environment
    (D) Deinstitutionalization

59. A client holds two opposing beliefs; one is that work is the most important thing in life and the second is that most enjoyment comes from leisure activities. Because this client feels this is a problem, the TRS might employ which of the following intervention techniques with this client?

    (A) Values clarification
    (B) Reality orientation
    (C) Remotivation
    (D) Cognitive restructuring

60. The TRS wants patients/clients with severe mental retardation to be able to freely choose their preferred leisure experiences. The TRS uses a variety of tactile, auditory, and gustatory objects during the use of which of the following intervention techniques?

    (A) Reality orientation
    (B) Remotivation
    (C) Assertiveness training
    (D) Sensory stimulation

61. Society generally devalues individuals with disabilities, reinforcing negative attitudes by doing which of the following:

    I.   Using offensive terminology with regard to people with disabilities
    II. Treating them as helpless and victimized
    III. Labeling them as social burdens

    (A) I and II only
    (B) I and III only
    (C) II and III only
    (D) I, II, and III

62. An adult with mental retardation has the ability to participate in some general recreation programs within the regular community-based recreation program. When the TRS helps the client enroll in one of these programs, which of the following mainstreaming principles is being applied?

    (A) Normalization
    (B) Deinstitutionalization
    (C) Least restrictive environment
    (D) Discharge planning

63. One of the most typical ways to receive direct reimbursement for TR services is by "time units." This means that the patient is charged

    (A) per time intervals (e.g., per 15 minutes)
    (B) as part of the per diem rate
    (C) by the procedures performed
    (D) by the hospital's daily bed rate

64. The TRS is working with teenagers in a psychiatric inpatient program that is oriented toward Freudian psychology. One of the activities the TRS would recommend for the clients based on "sublimation of sexual urges" is

    (A) crafts
    (B) a dance
    (C) gymnastics
    (D) tennis

65. Which of the following activities is MOST LIKELY to teach social skills to a group of at-risk youth?

    (A) Bingo
    (B) Volleyball, because it involves both cooperation and competition
    (C) Role plays of asking someone for assistance
    (D) Discussion of appropriate social skills in a variety of situations

66. Many private hospitals followed the federal government in adhering to a prospective payment system. This means that

    (A) hospitals receive the same fee for each diagnostic-related group (DRG) they treat
    (B) insurance companies will pay whatever hospitals charge for a service
    (C) individuals pay 80 percent of health care charges
    (D) psychiatric services are available to individuals within their own community

67. Charlie receives a token every time he responds appropriately to a request from a staff member. This therapy is called

    (A) behavior management
    (B) behavior modification
    (C) behavior therapy
    (D) milieu therapy

68. Which of the following is an example of using "displacement" as a defense mechanism?

    (A) Not remembering that the event occurred
    (B) Attributing the action or behavior to another person
    (C) Using a subordinate as the scapegoat
    (D) Not acknowledging the magnitude of a stressful event

69. Current research has shown that the most common TR services billed for reimbursement include

    (A) client assessment, leisure education, and community re-entry
    (B) client assessment, social skills training, and ADLs
    (C) stress management, group activities, and outpatient services
    (D) values clarification, leisure education, and functional skills training

70. A TRS is working with a group of adolescents who have mild mental retardation and hopes to improve their interactions with each other. She has decided to use positive reinforcement for each good interaction that occurs with the group. The first thing the TRS should do is

    (A) determine how often the target behavior currently occurs
    (B) determine what is a reinforcer
    (C) reward each client whenever a good interaction occurs
    (D) describe the target behavior

71. In a facility that adopts the Health Protection/Health Promotion model, what is the primary purpose of the intervention?

    (A) To provide therapist-directed experiences with clients
    (B) To motivate clients to function independently in the community
    (C) To promote behaviors that enable clients to move toward mastery of their own health
    (D) To enhance leisure decision-making so clients develop self and leisure awareness

72. The medical term "oriented x3" is the abbreviation for

    (A) can go as high as 3 times tables in math skills
    (B) recognizes 3 objects
    (C) oriented to person, place and time
    (D) can have three visitors at a time

73. The medical term "qid" is the abbreviation for

    (A) white blood count
    (B) four times a day
    (C) quadriceps
    (D) within normal limits

74. In order for a person to be nationally certified, by the National Council for Therapeutic Recreation Certification, at the C.T.R.S.-professional level (academic path), which of the following fieldwork requirements must be met?

    (A) The on-site fieldwork supervisor must be a C.T.R.S.
    (B) The university supervisor must be a C.T.R.S.
    (C) A 15-week fieldwork requirement must be completed.
    (D) The fieldwork placement must be completed at two different agencies (clinical and community).

75. The major difference between an acute care hospital and a physical rehabilitation center is the

    (A) types of professionals found on the treatment team
    (B) patient's/client's readiness for outpatient programs
    (C) patient's/client's medical stability and need for care
    (D) level of professional accountability required by external accreditation standards

76. The TRS evaluated the 16-week summer programming sessions at four-week, eight-week, and twelve-week intervals to gather which of the following types of program evaluation information?

    (A) Instantaneous time sampling
    (B) Quality assurance health care monitoring
    (C) Formative
    (D) Summative

77. Which of the following would be typical topics for specific program evaluation questions?

    (A) Content of the assessment and content of the program
    (B) Seasonal program offerings and timing of events
    (C) Validity and reliability of the specific program evaluation questions
    (D) Appropriateness of program content and process for clients who participated

78. A TRS is looking for program ideas for adolescent chemical abusers. The BEST resource for the TRS is

    (A) the Therapeutic Recreation Journal
    (B) state recreation conferences
    (C) chemical dependence conference
    (D) other therapeutic recreation professionals who work in chemical dependency

79. In what document would the TRS be MOST likely to find information on staff benefits?

    (A) Quality improvement records
    (B) Policy and procedure manual
    (C) Intern manual
    (D) Personnel files

80. The term "continuity of care" means that the

    (A) treatment team strives to provide predictable, connected, meaningful programs to clients
    (B) client is transitioned from clinical to community settings
    (C) client is involved in inclusive recreation services in the community with non-disabled peers
    (D) specialist serves as a case manager throughout the client's length of stay at the facility

81. The purpose of quality improvement activities is to

    (A) gather client input into the improvement of programs
    (B) increase communication with other members of the treatment team
    (C) increase documentation of therapeutic recreation services
    (D) improve the effectiveness of client services

82. Which of the following agencies is responsible for developing standards for facilities that serve individuals with spinal cord injuries, chronic pain, and traumatic brain injuries?

    (A) American Therapeutic Recreation Association (ATRA)
    (B) Joint Commission on Accreditation of Healthcare Organizations (JCAHO)
    (C) Centers for Medicare and Medicaid Services (CMS)
    (D) Rehabilitation Accreditation Commission (CARF)

83. The primary role of therapeutic recreation specialists working with individuals who have autism is to

    (A) have them learn a variety of leisure skills that their peers might know
    (B) promote independent functioning to the greatest extent possible
    (C) teach them how to adapt to a non-autistic world
    (D) learn leisure skills that they can use as teenagers and young adults

Question 84

84. Consider the following statements when answering question 84.

    I.   Assessments must be selected or developed based on a specific purpose.
    II. Assessments must be able to gather necessary information in a logical and straightforward manner.
    III. Assessments must meet the needs of the clients and intent of the agency.
    IV. Assessments must be able to produce results that are valid and reliable to the greatest degree possible.

    Which of these are true statements about client assessment in therapeutic recreation?

    (A) I only
    (B) II and III only
    (C) II, III, and IV only
    (D) I, II, III, and IV

85. In systems program design, a performance measure (PM) is the same as a(n)

    (A) assessment item
    (B) outcome statement
    (C) enabling objective
    (D) mission statement

86. If the therapeutic recreation specialist makes an error while writing in Thelma's chart, he should

    (A) use white correction fluid over the error and then write the correction in ink
    (B) report the mistake to his boss, and begin on a clean new page
    (C) cross out the error, write "error" above it and initial it
    (D) learn to always chart in pencil so mistakes can easily be erased and corrected

87. Tammy is asked to submit an annual budget that assumes she starts with no dollars and asks her to justify each dollar she then requests. This type of budgeting is called

    (A) zero-based budgeting
    (B) zero-sum score budgeting
    (C) revenue and expense budgeting
    (D) NIL (No Income or Losses) budgeting

88. After each out-trip the therapeutic recreation specialist is required to perform an 11-point checklist on the van. What is the purpose of this task?

    (A) Vehicle inspection
    (B) Quality improvement
    (C) Vehicle evaluation
    (D) Risk management

89. Once Carlinda has met the sitting requirements for and passed the NCTRC exam, she must renew her certification every _____ years(s) and recertify every _____ year(s) to remain certified.

    (A) five, ten
    (B) one, five
    (C) two, six
    (D) one, two

90. Liang is aware that clients, like the rest of the American population, are apt to be more overweight and obese as they are admitted, and he realizes this puts them at risk of not having a healthy and satisfying leisure lifestyle. To find out information about this trend as well as ways to reverse it, Liang should read documents at which of the following web sites?

    (A) www.toofatforhealth.org
    (B) www.healthypeople.gov
    (C) www.takebackyourtime.org
    (D) www.recreationtherapy.com

Practice Test 1
Scoring Sheet

1. Ⓐ Ⓑ Ⓒ Ⓓ   14. Ⓐ Ⓑ Ⓒ Ⓓ   27. Ⓐ Ⓑ Ⓒ Ⓓ   40. Ⓐ Ⓑ Ⓒ Ⓓ

2. Ⓐ Ⓑ Ⓒ Ⓓ   15. Ⓐ Ⓑ Ⓒ Ⓓ   28. Ⓐ Ⓑ Ⓒ Ⓓ   41. Ⓐ Ⓑ Ⓒ Ⓓ

3. Ⓐ Ⓑ Ⓒ Ⓓ   16. Ⓐ Ⓑ Ⓒ Ⓓ   29. Ⓐ Ⓑ Ⓒ Ⓓ   42. Ⓐ Ⓑ Ⓒ Ⓓ

4. Ⓐ Ⓑ Ⓒ Ⓓ   17. Ⓐ Ⓑ Ⓒ Ⓓ   30. Ⓐ Ⓑ Ⓒ Ⓓ   43. Ⓐ Ⓑ Ⓒ Ⓓ

5. Ⓐ Ⓑ Ⓒ Ⓓ   18. Ⓐ Ⓑ Ⓒ Ⓓ   31. Ⓐ Ⓑ Ⓒ Ⓓ   44. Ⓐ Ⓑ Ⓒ Ⓓ

6. Ⓐ Ⓑ Ⓒ Ⓓ   19. Ⓐ Ⓑ Ⓒ Ⓓ   32. Ⓐ Ⓑ Ⓒ Ⓓ   45. Ⓐ Ⓑ Ⓒ Ⓓ

7. Ⓐ Ⓑ Ⓒ Ⓓ   20. Ⓐ Ⓑ Ⓒ Ⓓ   33. Ⓐ Ⓑ Ⓒ Ⓓ   46. Ⓐ Ⓑ Ⓒ Ⓓ

8. Ⓐ Ⓑ Ⓒ Ⓓ   21. Ⓐ Ⓑ Ⓒ Ⓓ   34. Ⓐ Ⓑ Ⓒ Ⓓ   47. Ⓐ Ⓑ Ⓒ Ⓓ

9. Ⓐ Ⓑ Ⓒ Ⓓ   22. Ⓐ Ⓑ Ⓒ Ⓓ   35. Ⓐ Ⓑ Ⓒ Ⓓ   48. Ⓐ Ⓑ Ⓒ Ⓓ

10. Ⓐ Ⓑ Ⓒ Ⓓ   23. Ⓐ Ⓑ Ⓒ Ⓓ   36. Ⓐ Ⓑ Ⓒ Ⓓ   49. Ⓐ Ⓑ Ⓒ Ⓓ

11. Ⓐ Ⓑ Ⓒ Ⓓ   24. Ⓐ Ⓑ Ⓒ Ⓓ   37. Ⓐ Ⓑ Ⓒ Ⓓ   50. Ⓐ Ⓑ Ⓒ Ⓓ

12. Ⓐ Ⓑ Ⓒ Ⓓ   25. Ⓐ Ⓑ Ⓒ Ⓓ   38. Ⓐ Ⓑ Ⓒ Ⓓ   51. Ⓐ Ⓑ Ⓒ Ⓓ

13. Ⓐ Ⓑ Ⓒ Ⓓ   26. Ⓐ Ⓑ Ⓒ Ⓓ   39. Ⓐ Ⓑ Ⓒ Ⓓ   52. Ⓐ Ⓑ Ⓒ Ⓓ

Practice Test 1
Scoring Sheet

53. Ⓐ Ⓑ Ⓒ Ⓓ   66. Ⓐ Ⓑ Ⓒ Ⓓ   79. Ⓐ Ⓑ Ⓒ Ⓓ

54. Ⓐ Ⓑ Ⓒ Ⓓ   67. Ⓐ Ⓑ Ⓒ Ⓓ   80. Ⓐ Ⓑ Ⓒ Ⓓ

55. Ⓐ Ⓑ Ⓒ Ⓓ   68. Ⓐ Ⓑ Ⓒ Ⓓ   81. Ⓐ Ⓑ Ⓒ Ⓓ

56. Ⓐ Ⓑ Ⓒ Ⓓ   69. Ⓐ Ⓑ Ⓒ Ⓓ   82. Ⓐ Ⓑ Ⓒ Ⓓ

57. Ⓐ Ⓑ Ⓒ Ⓓ   70. Ⓐ Ⓑ Ⓒ Ⓓ   83. Ⓐ Ⓑ Ⓒ Ⓓ

58. Ⓐ Ⓑ Ⓒ Ⓓ   71. Ⓐ Ⓑ Ⓒ Ⓓ   84. Ⓐ Ⓑ Ⓒ Ⓓ

59. Ⓐ Ⓑ Ⓒ Ⓓ   72. Ⓐ Ⓑ Ⓒ Ⓓ   85. Ⓐ Ⓑ Ⓒ Ⓓ

60. Ⓐ Ⓑ Ⓒ Ⓓ   73. Ⓐ Ⓑ Ⓒ Ⓓ   86. Ⓐ Ⓑ Ⓒ Ⓓ

61. Ⓐ Ⓑ Ⓒ Ⓓ   74. Ⓐ Ⓑ Ⓒ Ⓓ   87. Ⓐ Ⓑ Ⓒ Ⓓ

62. Ⓐ Ⓑ Ⓒ Ⓓ   75. Ⓐ Ⓑ Ⓒ Ⓓ   88. Ⓐ Ⓑ Ⓒ Ⓓ

63. Ⓐ Ⓑ Ⓒ Ⓓ   76. Ⓐ Ⓑ Ⓒ Ⓓ   89. Ⓐ Ⓑ Ⓒ Ⓓ

64. Ⓐ Ⓑ Ⓒ Ⓓ   77. Ⓐ Ⓑ Ⓒ Ⓓ   90. Ⓐ Ⓑ Ⓒ Ⓓ

65. Ⓐ Ⓑ Ⓒ Ⓓ   78. Ⓐ Ⓑ Ⓒ Ⓓ

Practice Test 1
Scoring Key

Background

1. **B**	11. **C**	12. **A**	13. **D**	32. **B**	71. **C**	75. **C**

Diagnostic Groupings

8. **A**	14. **A**	16. **B**	19. **D**	20. **B**	30. **D**	
31. **A**	33. **B**	35. **A**	36. **C**	37. **C**	83. **B**	

Assessment

6. **B**	9. **D**	10. **A**	17. **A**	21. **C**	25. **A**	40. **D**
43. **B**	44. **C**	48. **C**	50. **D**	51. **C**	52. **B**	55. **B**
84. **D**						

Planning the Intervention

3. **B**	4. **D**	22. **B**	23. **C**	27. **D**	34. **B**	41. **A**
42. **A**	53. **C**	54. **D**	58. **B**	61. **D**	62. **A**	85. **B**

Implementing the Individual Intervention Plan

2. **D**	15. **D**	18. **C**	24. **B**	26. **A**	38. **B**	39. **C**
59. **A**	60. **D**	64. **B**	65. **C**	67. **B**	68. **C**	70. **D**

Documentation and Evaluation

7. **C**	45. **C**	46. **D**	56. **D**	57. **A**	63. **A**	69. **A**
72. **C**	73. **B**	76. **C**	77. **D**	79. **B**	80. **A**	86. **C**

Organizing and Managing Services

28. **B**	29. **C**	47. **C**	66. **A**	81. **D**	82. **D**	87. **A**
88. **D**						

Advancement of the Profession

5. **B**	49. **C**	74. **A**	78. **D**	89. **B**	90. **B**

Record Your Scores Here:

Background   ____/ 7 = ____ %
Diagnostic Groupings   ____/13 = ____ %
Assessment   ____/14 = ____ %
Planning the Intervention   ____/14 = ____ %
Implementing the Intervention   ____/14 = ____ %
Documenting/Evaluation   ____/14 = ____ %
Organizing/Managing   ____/ 8 = ____ %
Advancement of the Profession   ____/ 6 = ____ %

Total Score   ____/90

Total Percent   ____ %

If you need more practice in any area(s), proceed to Practice Test 2.

Practice Test 2

The sample questions that follow represent the types of questions included in the NCTRC Certification Exam. The purpose of this Practice Test is to give you some indication of how it will feel to take the actual NCTRC exam. The length of the test, and content and format of the questions is close to that of the national test.

Directions: For each question in this section, select the best of the answer choices given. Use the answer sheet on page 130 to record your answers. Use the scoring key on page 132 to score your answers.

---

1. The basis for behavioristic theory comes from

    (A) understanding the hidden unconscious forces that underlie behavior
    (B) examining a person's thinking process and the effects of those thoughts on behaviors and emotions
    (C) academic learning theory
    (D) making people focus on reality

2. To receive the full benefits of a leisure experience, most TRSs believe that the experience should be

    (A) spontaneous
    (B) motivational
    (C) intrinsically motivated
    (D) challenging

3. One of the primary criteria for selecting client assessments for use in therapeutic recreation programs is that

    (A) the content of the assessment matches the content of the intervention program
    (B) it improves the expertise of the specialist
    (C) the inter-rater reliability is high
    (D) it requires specialized training just for therapeutic recreation specialists

4. Aging women, as compared to men, are cared for in long-term care facilities at the rate of

    (A) 4 women to 3 men
    (B) 10 women to 9 men
    (C) 1 woman to 2 men
    (D) 2 women to 1 man

Question 5

The most widely used therapeutic recreation service model consists of the three areas of service provision listed below. Select the one that BEST fits each of the following goal statements.

    I. Functional Intervention
   II. Leisure Education
  III. Recreation Participation

5. To seek life balance by participating in "fun" activities while in the facility

    (A) I only
    (B) II only
    (C) III only
    (D) I and III only

6. The medical term "VO" is the abbreviation for

    (A) verbal order
    (B) halitosis
    (C) ventilator only
    (D) vital organism

7. All of the following have an impact on how client documentation is recorded, EXCEPT:

    (A) external accreditation standards
    (B) agency guidelines and procedures
    (C) legal requirements
    (D) professional development

8. The TRS can make which of the following assumptions about clients in a day care center for older adults?

    (A) They are in need of acute medical care.
    (B) They have or can arrange transportation and have a reasonable level of health.
    (C) They live below the income poverty level.
    (D) They need reality orientation and remotivation training activities.

9. For individuals with disabilities, beginning at age 14, a transition plan for services must be in place, as required by what piece of federal legislation?

    (A) Rehabilitation Act of 1978
    (B) Americans with Disabilities Act of 1990
    (C) New Freedom Initiative of 2000
    (D) Individuals with Disabilities Education Act of 1997

10. The definition of mental retardation adopted by the American Association of Mental Deficiency (AAMD) suggests that there is a relationship between mental functioning and which of the following?

    (A) Social skills
    (B) Physical skills
    (C) Lability
    (D) Adaptive behavior

Questions 11-13

    I. Assessment
   II. Program Planning
  III. Program Implementation
  IV. Program Evaluation

Match the action given below in each question with the appropriate step of program planning above.

11. This action taken by the specialist requires an examination of how the content and process of the activity will contribute to the accomplishment of client objectives

    (A) I only
    (B) II only
    (C) I, II, and III only
    (D) I, II, III, and IV

12. This action taken by the specialist allows the client to be placed into the most appropriate program to meet his or her needs

    (A) I only
    (B) II only
    (C) I, II, and III only
    (D) I, II, III, and IV

13. This action taken by the specialist provides feedback for the future improvement of programs

    (A) I only
    (B) II only
    (C) IV only
    (D) I, II, III, and IV

14. Persons who demonstrate enduring, maladaptive patterns of relating to, perceiving, and thinking about the environment and themselves causing significant impairment of social or occupational functioning or subjective distress are considered to have which of the following disorders?

    (A) Anxiety
    (B) Personality
    (C) Affective
    (D) Schizophrenic

15. When using active listening with a client, it is important for the TRS to do which of the following?

    (A) Reflect the feeling tone the client communicates
    (B) Respond immediately to the client's statements
    (C) Nod his/her head and speak to the client frequently
    (D) Ask questions so the client will know the TRS is listening

16. One of the MOST important aspects of a client/therapist relationship is for the TRS to

    (A) have an unconditional positive regard for the client
    (B) let the client know he/she is always right
    (C) establish a position of authority with the client
    (D) establish a relationship with the client's family

17. A TRS is working with a person who is a quadriplegic as a result of a recent diving accident. The TRS suggests that she try playing ping-pong instead of tennis, which she has previously enjoyed. The TRS is using which of the following therapeutic recreation principles?

    I. Social integration
    II. Substitutability
    III. Least restrictive environment

    (A) I only
    (B) II only
    (C) II and III only
    (D) I, II, and III

18. Which of the following would improve the reliability of the results of an assessment tool?

    (A) Replace all closed-ended items with open-ended items
    (B) Shorten the length of the assessment
    (C) Remove all items that were ambiguous to the clients
    (D) Limit the time the client has to complete the assessment

19. Asking the question, "How stable is the instrument over a given period of time?" is an example of looking at the assessment's

    (A) concurrent validity statistics
    (B) test-retest estimates
    (C) Cronbach's alpha
    (D) internal consistency estimates

20. The specialist says to the client, during a therapeutic recreation program, "Let's stay in the present and take responsibility for your actions." This specialist is using which type of "therapy" approach?

    (A) Gestalt therapy
    (B) Rational-emotive therapy
    (C) Cognitive therapy
    (D) Reality therapy

21. When a person experiences stress, which of the following physiological reactions occur?

    (A) blood pressure lowers
    (B) pupils (eyes) become dilated
    (C) respirations decrease
    (D) blood rushes to the hands and feet

22. Typical characteristics of violent youth include

    (A) low self-esteem, lack of empathy, and low frustration tolerance
    (B) high socioeconomic status, lack of anger management, and impulsivity
    (C) low self-esteem, high self-control, and low frustration tolerance
    (D) high stress tolerance, lack of empathy, and low socioeconomic status

23. One of the problems with client assessment in therapeutic recreation services is that

    (A) there are too many assessments from which to select
    (B) clients are too diverse to be assessed
    (C) assessments that are validated for practice are difficult to find and use
    (D) the information they gather is often in conflict with that of other treatment team members

24. Which of the following is MOST likely to produce positive attitudes toward individuals with disabilities?

    (A) Increased exposure and contact to individuals with disabilities
    (B) Special discount rates to events and attractions
    (C) Segregated or specialized services for individuals with disabilities
    (D) Negative terminology and extensive classification systems

25. The TRS working in a psychiatric facility for adults needs an assessment instrument that has the capability of monitoring clients in the three areas of general performance, individual performance, and group performance. Which of the following published assessment instruments would be MOST suitable?

    (A) Leisure Diagnostic Battery (LDB)
    (B) Comprehensive Evaluation in Recreational Therapy Scale (CERT)
    (C) Self-Leisure Interest Profile (SLIP)
    (D) Leisure Activities Blank (LAB)

26. Which of the following individuals likely has cataracts?

    (A) Kia needs glasses only for near-vision reading.
    (B) Alfred experiences loss of central vision and has to turn from side to side to see an item directly in front of him.
    (C) Sophie's vision is blurred and she has trouble seeing things distinctly.
    (D) Colletta has difficulty seeing at night, often seeing "stars" around bright lights.

27. Mental illness may be considered any disorder that

    (A) is congenital and transient
    (B) results from lower intellectual capacity and lower adaptive behavior
    (C) results in abnormal behavior that can be seen as bizarre, unusual, and irritating
    (D) exhibits alteration of thought, mood or behavior so that the individual has difficulty meeting daily living requirements

28. The client's goal is to develop appropriate competitive skills. The therapist selects table games like checkers and tic tac toe to initiate intervention. At what social interaction level has the TRS begun intervention?

    (A) Extra individual
    (B) Aggregate
    (C) Inter-individual
    (D) Unilateral

29. The TRS places a client in a team sport to introduce cognitive challenges. What higher level intellectual requirement is needed to be successful in a team sport like soccer?

    (A) Memorization of rules
    (B) Coordination of body parts
    (C) Comprehension of the plays
    (D) Application of strategies

30. According to Maslow, all humans are striving to achieve _____ but first must fulfill other essential needs.

    (A) self-actualization
    (B) ego esteem needs
    (C) a sense of love and belonging
    (D) safety/security

31. When working with persons who are mentally retarded, the TRS should

    (A) present the activity in small steps
    (B) demonstrate when possible
    (C) move through activities quickly to keep their attention
    (D) A and B

32. Clyde was discharged from the clinical facility because it was determined that he was not making further progress in his rehabilitation efforts and the "bed space" could be better utilized for an incoming patient. Which of the following committees or departments would make this recommendation?

    (A) Professional standards review organization (PSRO)
    (B) Utilization review
    (C) Medical records review
    (D) Risk management review

33. Which of the following is NOT appropriate to document in the therapeutic recreation department's written plan of operation?

    (A) The philosophy of the therapeutic recreation department
    (B) Comprehensive and specific program descriptions
    (C) The description of assessment tool and procedures
    (D) The treatment plans and progress notes

34. Paralysis on one side of the body is called

    (A) paraplegia
    (B) hemiplegia
    (C) monoplegia
    (D) quadriplegia

35. Hazel is showing signs of disorientation, confusion and memory loss. After the TRS completes the assessment and meets with the treatment team, he/she should use which of the following intervention techniques?

    (A) Resocialization
    (B) Remotivation
    (C) Reality orientation
    (D) Refocusing

36. The TRS designed a program to assist older adults with mental retardation to share their past life experiences after reading poetry about children. The TRS was using a technique known as _____ .

    (A) reality orientation
    (B) remotivation
    (C) resocialization
    (D) cognitive restructuring

37. The specialist employs an activity that focuses on the client's thoughts. What is this kind of therapy called?

    (A) Cognitive therapy
    (B) Behavior therapy
    (C) Affective therapy
    (D) Gestalt therapy

38. A TRS wants to assess a patient's/client's ability to control anger. The TRS should assess behavior from which of the following domains?

    (A) Cognitive
    (B) Physical
    (C) Emotional
    (D) Social

39. If a facility does not meet standards and is not accredited by the Joint Commission on Accreditation of Healthcare Organizations (JCAHO), what is likely to be the result?

    (A) Medicare, Medicaid, and private insurance companies will not pay for services.
    (B) The administration will seek accreditation by CARF.
    (C) Staff's wages will be garnished until the problem is corrected.
    (D) Nothing, accreditation by the Joint Commission is not mandatory.

40. An individual's responses or scores on the Minimum Data Set (MDS) may link to a "trigger" that requires a Resident Assessment Protocol (RAP) to be completed. This means that

    (A) an individual will receive a more in-depth assessment in this area
    (B) the TRS must complete an interview with the family
    (C) the assessment was completed incorrectly
    (D) the information from the assessment is neither valid or reliable

41. Which of the following is NOT criteria for selecting "important aspects of care" to monitor during quality assurance reviews?

    (A) Programs that serve large numbers of clients
    (B) Programs that put clients at risk of serious consequences
    (C) Programs that occur on an annual basis
    (D) Programs that, in the past, have produced problems for staff or clients

42. Which of the following is the BEST example of an efficacy research study conducted in a physical rehabilitation setting?

    (A) Client skills at discharge are compared with their skills at admission
    (B) The TRS tracks client attendance at therapeutic recreation programs
    (C) Two TRSs evaluate the inter-rater reliability of their observational assessment tool
    (D) Peer reviews are conducted on adherence to NTRS and ATRA *Standards of Practice*

43. When serving a program evaluation function, the assessment tool or procedure and its results may be used to

    (A) plan appropriate programs for client needs
    (B) provide an accurate and valid diagnosis for client treatment
    (C) monitor the continuing behavior of clients
    (D) ask for input from the other therapists on the treatment team

44. While teaching adolescents with mild mental retardation the card game of "Hearts," the TRS found that she unexpectedly needed to repeat directions throughout the game. The TRS had inappropriately analyzed and planned the activity in which of the following domains?

    (A) Physical
    (B) Emotional
    (C) Social
    (D) Cognitive

45. What does the use of categorizing and labeling individuals with disabilities reflect?

    (A) Misconception about professionalism
    (B) Attitudes held toward individuals with disabilities
    (C) Inadequate information about health and illness
    (D) Religious beliefs toward perceived differences

46. All of the following things affect people's attitudes toward individuals with disabilities, EXCEPT:

    (A) characters portrayed in movies
    (B) fairy tales and childhood stories
    (C) etiological concerns
    (D) television advertisements

47. Which of the following assessments would be located in the category of Leisure Attitudes and Barriers?

    (A) Leisure Motivation Scale (LMS)
    (B) Ohio Scales of Leisure Functioning
    (C) Therapeutic Recreation Index (TRI)
    (D) Recreation Behavior Inventory (RBI)

Questions 48-51

      I. Intragroup
     II. Multilateral
    III. Interindividual
     IV. Extraindividual

Match one of the interaction patterns above, with the statement or activity below.

48. Most video games

    (A) I only
    (B) II only
    (C) III only
    (D) IV only

49. Most common adult social interaction pattern

    (A) I only
    (B) II only
    (C) III only
    (D) IV only

50. Action with an object in the environment, requires no contact with another person

    (A) I only
    (B) II only
    (C) III only
    (D) IV only

51. Singles tennis

    (A) I only
    (B) II only
    (C) III only
    (D) IV only

Questions 52-54

Several methods of observing and recording behavior can be used in assessment. Using the methods below, choose the appropriate observational method for the situation.

    I. Frequency
    II. Duration
    III. Latency
    IV. Time sampling

52. The TRS wants to know how long it takes a client to start a task when assigned.

    (A) I only
    (B) II only
    (C) III only
    (D) IV only

53. The TRS wants to know how many times a client refuses to attend therapeutic recreation programs.

    (A) I only
    (B) II only
    (C) III only
    (D) IV only

54. The TRS checks the activity room at 9:00, 11:00, 1:00 and 3:00 to see how many patients are watching television.

    (A) I only
    (B) II only
    (C) III only
    (D) IV only

55. When a TRS provides an accepting and understanding attitude to a client and, as a result, that positive involvement reduces the client's feelings of loneliness and worthlessness, and helps the client to take responsibility to alter irresponsible behavior, the TRS is probably using _____ therapy.

    (A) psychoanalytic
    (B) behavior
    (C) reality
    (D) rational emotive

56. A TRS is nonjudgmental, nondirective, and provides an accepting atmosphere allowing the client to assume the same positive self-regard the TRS has shown to the client. The TRS is using _____ .

    (A) gestalt
    (B) reality
    (C) rational emotive
    (D) person centered

57. When a physician or case manager creates a master list of client deficits and develops a plan of action focused on these deficits, this is called

    (A) a problem-oriented medical record
    (B) the number of clients served on the unit and space available
    (C) the case load of the physician on staff
    (D) the patient's needs and nature of the program

58. In the mental illness diagnosis classification system used by the American Psychiatric Association, Axes I and II describe

    (A) physical disorders related to mental illness
    (B) unrelated symptoms
    (C) categories and conditions of mental illness
    (D) social support networks that can be used by the client

59. One example of a mood disorder is the diagnosis of

    (A) psychosis
    (B) bipolar personality
    (C) paranoia
    (D) organic brain syndrome

60. In 1983, a cost-cutting Medicare hospital payment system was initiated that included

    (A) a retrospective payment system
    (B) direct reimbursement for therapeutic recreation services
    (C) the Centers for Medicare and Medicaid Services (CMS)
    (D) diagnostic-related groups (DRGs)

61. Which of the following statements represents an assertive response to the question "Where would you like to eat dinner tonight?"

    (A) "We can go wherever you want."
    (B) "I don't care where we eat, you always choose anyway."
    (C) "I'd like to try that new Italian restaurant by the mall."
    (D) "You should know where I want to eat by now."

62. During an assessment interview, the client stated, "I hate physical activities. They just wear me out. But my sister just loves to be involved in sports." The TRS responded, "You don't like exercise, while your sister does." The TRS was using which of the following communication techniques?

    (A) Probe
    (B) Summarization
    (C) Redirection
    (D) Confrontation

63. During a leisure planning session, a client said, "We used to take lots of vacations as a family, usually for two to three weeks at a time." The TRS responded, "Tell me more about your vacations." The TRS was using which of the following communication techniques?

    (A) Probe
    (B) Summarization
    (C) Clarification
    (D) Confrontation

64. Which of the following is an appropriate program evaluation question to ask clients?

    (A) How satisfied were you with the qualifications of the staff?
    (B) What did you learn from your participation in this program?
    (C) How do you spend your time with family?
    (D) How satisfied were you with the activity analysis of this program?

65. Which of the following professional organizations is a branch of the National Recreation and Park Association?

    (A) National Council for Therapeutic Recreation Certification (NCTRC)
    (B) American Therapeutic Recreation Association (ATRA)
    (C) National Therapeutic Recreation Society (NTRS)
    (D) Recreation Therapy Section (RTS)

66. What is the purpose of the Health Protection/Health Promotion Model?

    (A) Independent leisure functioning
    (B) Facilitating healthy self-actualization
    (C) Attaining highest level of health
    (D) Reducing blocks to quality of life behaviors

67. During a leisure education discussion group, Peter sits slumped in his chair with his arms folded and legs crossed. Using non-verbal communication cues, the TRS assumes that Peter is

    (A) actively engaged in the activity
    (B) becoming overtly aggressive to other patients/clients
    (C) disinterested and unengaged in the activity
    (D) demonstrating a "closed" position to further communication

68. Which question below addresses client evaluation?

    (A) How consistent are the services being delivered to clients?
    (B) How many programs did the client attend?
    (C) Was the specialist effective and efficient in delivering intervention services to the client?
    (D) What proposed outcomes were achieved as the result of the client's involvement in the program?

69. Which of the following is an example of "objective" data that may be recorded in a progress note?

    (A) The client stated, "I really got a lot out of this program!".
    (B) The client's family said that the client was progressing with the outpatient therapy.
    (C) The client interacted with a peer for two minutes, discussing the role of leisure in their lives.
    (D) The client appears depressed and withdrawn after counseling sessions.

70. Which of the following is the BEST example of a client outcome measure, collected as part of the therapeutic recreation department's quality improvement efforts?

    (A) Change in clients' health status or well-being
    (B) Change in client's attendance at programs
    (C) Development of a baseline for expected client behavior
    (D) Development of one-to-one treatment programs

71. A written plan of operation for a therapeutic recreation department is a

    (A) policy and procedure manual
    (B) description of the department's quality performance initiatives
    (C) personnel maintenance record
    (D) summary of all departmental risk management activities for the past five years

Questions 72 - 75

Select from the elements of the SOAP progress note the one that BEST fits each of the following.

    I. Schedule pt. for social interaction program.
    II. Patient turns away when others try to talk with him/her and attends to a craft or a book.
    III. Patient refuses to talk in a social situation to hospital staff or other patients although he/she has been observed talking to family members.
    IV. Patient states: "Don't bother me."

72. The plan

    (A) I only
    (B) II only
    (C) III only
    (D) IV only

73. The subjective data

    (A) I only
    (B) II only
    (C) III only
    (D) IV only

74. The objective data

    (A) I only
    (B) II only
    (C) III only
    (D) IV only

75. The assessment data

    (A) I only
    (B) II only
    (C) III only
    (D) IV only

76. As the level of mental retardation increases from mild to severe/profound, the TRS should expect to see increased

    (A) social and intellectual skill development
    (B) compensation for skill deficits
    (C) need for transportation
    (D) secondary physical limitations and sensory impairments

77. If a client receives treatment and was not informed of risks involved and the treatment results in some unwanted side effect or injury, then the client can bring a lawsuit against the TRS. The TRS could be found

    (A) guilty of negligence
    (B) having a breach of confidentiality
    (C) to be harmful to all
    (D) guilty of malfeasance

78. In a facility that utilizes the medical model of services, the TRS would focus on which of the following?

    (A) The patient's/client's problem or pathology related to leisure
    (B) Providing activities and games which promote physical development
    (C) Integrating the patient/client into ongoing community recreation programs
    (D) Documenting critical incidents of the patient's/client's medical stability

79. According to the World Health Organization's International Classification of Functioning, Disability, and Health (ICF), services are needed at each of the following levels:

    (A) Community, state, regional, and national
    (B) Body part, the whole person, and the person's social context
    (C) Medical, rehabilitation, and long-term care
    (D) Functional intervention, leisure education, and recreation participation

80. Bart organizes his therapeutic recreation department so that the focus is on client outcomes that are systematically determined, intentional, change-oriented, and controlled for. His department is aiming at _____.

    (A) holistic health
    (B) intervention
    (C) health promotion
    (D) health recovery

81. Sybil uses the Transtheoretical Model of Behavior change in organizing her documentation on client behavior change. What are the "stages" of behavior change that Sybil observes and documents on?

    (A) Thought, affect, behavior, evaluation
    (B) Rapid behavior change, slowed behavior change, and maintained behavior change
    (C) Precontemplation, contemplation, preparation, action, maintenance, and termination
    (D) Preparation, action, evaluation, and new action

82. Which of the following are typical parts of a client treatment plan?

    (A) Assessment results, goals and objectives, interventions, and reevaluation schedule
    (B) Client deficits, statements, behaviors, and plans for change
    (C) Current status, past status, and future status
    (D) Strengths, plan of action, and plan for re-evaluation

83. Units or facilities that are especially designed for individuals with moderate to advanced dementia include which of the following design considerations?

    (A) Mazes for wandering, bright colors, no signage, heavy security doors
    (B) Minimal clutter, no more than 10 residents per unit, one large bedroom for all 10
    (C) Clusters of residences, meaningful wandering path, positive and secure outdoor space
    (D) Walking paths through the community, well-lit areas, large activity spaces

84. Which of the following is a question that addresses content validity?

    (A) How accurately does current content reflect future content?
    (B) How closely related are items on a single assessment?
    (C) How consistent are scores over different parts of the assessment?
    (D) How adequately does the sample of assessment items represent the totality of the content to be measured?

85. Chia received burns in a house fire that affected all three layers of skin as well as muscle tissue. She does not feel pain as the nerve fibers and pain receptors have been destroyed. Chia's burns are classified as

    (A) intensive
    (B) first-degree
    (C) second-degree
    (D) third-degree

86. Cherise bases her intervention programs on the notion that all clients desire to interact effectively with their physical and social environments and to view themselves as skilled in their quest for a happy and fulfilling life. She is basing her intervention programs on the theory of

    (A) competence-effectance motivation
    (B) trust-building
    (C) self-determination
    (D) social psychology of leisure

87. Edy requires that all of her employees actively participate in diversity training on a regular basis. She is trying to ensure their _____.

    (A) prejudices
    (B) cultural competence
    (C) attitudinal awareness
    (D) recertification through NCTRC

88. Kahlil wants to develop a stress management program. He first reviews the *Therapeutic Recreation Journal,* the *Annual in Therapeutic Recreation,* and the *American Journal of Recreation Therapy* to determine what is known about the design and effects of stress management programs in therapeutic recreation. Kahlil is performing what task?

    (A) A literature review
    (B) A research study
    (C) Evidence-based practice
    (D) A meta-analysis

89. Which of the following is NOT likely to aid a TRS in assessing his or her own competence?

    (A) NTRS's Standards of Practice
    (B) ATRA's Standards of Practice and Self-Assessment Guide
    (C) NCTRC's certification examination
    (D) Joint Commission's Comprehensive Accreditation Manual for Hospitals

90. Which of the following are NOT minimal expectations of all therapeutic recreation specialists?

    (A) Read professional journals, attend professional conferences, and network
    (B) Retain professional certification and join appropriate professional organizations
    (C) Study external accreditation documents and professional standards
    (D) Maintain professional knowledge as it was at graduation

Practice Test 2 Items
Answer Scoring Sheet

1. (A) (B) (C) (D)   14. (A) (B) (C) (D)   27. (A) (B) (C) (D)   40. (A) (B) (C) (D)

2. (A) (B) (C) (D)   15. (A) (B) (C) (D)   28. (A) (B) (C) (D)   41. (A) (B) (C) (D)

3. (A) (B) (C) (D)   16. (A) (B) (C) (D)   29. (A) (B) (C) (D)   42. (A) (B) (C) (D)

4. (A) (B) (C) (D)   17. (A) (B) (C) (D)   30. (A) (B) (C) (D)   43. (A) (B) (C) (D)

5. (A) (B) (C) (D)   18. (A) (B) (C) (D)   31. (A) (B) (C) (D)   44. (A) (B) (C) (D)

6. (A) (B) (C) (D)   19. (A) (B) (C) (D)   32. (A) (B) (C) (D)   45. (A) (B) (C) (D)

7. (A) (B) (C) (D)   20. (A) (B) (C) (D)   33. (A) (B) (C) (D)   46. (A) (B) (C) (D)

8. (A) (B) (C) (D)   21. (A) (B) (C) (D)   34. (A) (B) (C) (D)   47. (A) (B) (C) (D)

9. (A) (B) (C) (D)   22. (A) (B) (C) (D)   35. (A) (B) (C) (D)   48. (A) (B) (C) (D)

10. (A) (B) (C) (D)   23. (A) (B) (C) (D)   36. (A) (B) (C) (D)   49. (A) (B) (C) (D)

11. (A) (B) (C) (D)   24. (A) (B) (C) (D)   37. (A) (B) (C) (D)   50. (A) (B) (C) (D)

12. (A) (B) (C) (D)   25. (A) (B) (C) (D)   38. (A) (B) (C) (D)   51. (A) (B) (C) (D)

13. (A) (B) (C) (D)   26. (A) (B) (C) (D)   39. (A) (B) (C) (D)   52. (A) (B) (C) (D)

53. Ⓐ Ⓑ Ⓒ Ⓓ   66. Ⓐ Ⓑ Ⓒ Ⓓ   79. Ⓐ Ⓑ Ⓒ Ⓓ

54. Ⓐ Ⓑ Ⓒ Ⓓ   67. Ⓐ Ⓑ Ⓒ Ⓓ   80. Ⓐ Ⓑ Ⓒ Ⓓ

55. Ⓐ Ⓑ Ⓒ Ⓓ   68. Ⓐ Ⓑ Ⓒ Ⓓ   81. Ⓐ Ⓑ Ⓒ Ⓓ

56. Ⓐ Ⓑ Ⓒ Ⓓ   69. Ⓐ Ⓑ Ⓒ Ⓓ   82. Ⓐ Ⓑ Ⓒ Ⓓ

57. Ⓐ Ⓑ Ⓒ Ⓓ   70. Ⓐ Ⓑ Ⓒ Ⓓ   83. Ⓐ Ⓑ Ⓒ Ⓓ

58. Ⓐ Ⓑ Ⓒ Ⓓ   71. Ⓐ Ⓑ Ⓒ Ⓓ   84. Ⓐ Ⓑ Ⓒ Ⓓ

59. Ⓐ Ⓑ Ⓒ Ⓓ   72. Ⓐ Ⓑ Ⓒ Ⓓ   85. Ⓐ Ⓑ Ⓒ Ⓓ

60. Ⓐ Ⓑ Ⓒ Ⓓ   73. Ⓐ Ⓑ Ⓒ Ⓓ   86. Ⓐ Ⓑ Ⓒ Ⓓ

61. Ⓐ Ⓑ Ⓒ Ⓓ   74. Ⓐ Ⓑ Ⓒ Ⓓ   87. Ⓐ Ⓑ Ⓒ Ⓓ

62. Ⓐ Ⓑ Ⓒ Ⓓ   75. Ⓐ Ⓑ Ⓒ Ⓓ   88. Ⓐ Ⓑ Ⓒ Ⓓ

63. Ⓐ Ⓑ Ⓒ Ⓓ   76. Ⓐ Ⓑ Ⓒ Ⓓ   89. Ⓐ Ⓑ Ⓒ Ⓓ

64. Ⓐ Ⓑ Ⓒ Ⓓ   77. Ⓐ Ⓑ Ⓒ Ⓓ   90. Ⓐ Ⓑ Ⓒ Ⓓ

65. Ⓐ Ⓑ Ⓒ Ⓓ   78. Ⓐ Ⓑ Ⓒ Ⓓ

Practice Test 2
Scoring Key

Background

| 2. | C | 5. | C | 8. | B | 17. | B | 30. | A | 66. | C | 77. | D |
| 78. | A | 86. | A |

Diagnostic Groupings

| 4. | A | 10. | D | 14. | B | 22. | A | 26. | C | 27. | D |
| 31. | D | 34. | B | 58. | C | 59. | B | 76. | D | 83. | C | 85. | D |

Assessment

| 3. | A | 18. | C | 19. | B | 23. | C | 25. | B | 38. | C | 40. | A |
| 43. | C | 47. | A | 52. | C | 53. | A | 54. | D | 84. | D |

Planning the Intervention

| 11. | B | 12. | A | 13. | C | 24. | A | 28. | C | 29. | D | 44. | D |
| 45. | B | 46. | C | 48. | D | 49. | B | 50. | D | 51. | C | 82. | A |

Implementing the Individual Intervention Plan

| 1. | C | 15. | A | 16. | A | 20. | D | 21. | B | 35. | C | 36. | B |
| 37. | A | 55. | C | 56. | D | 61. | C | 62. | B | 63. | A | 67. | D |

Documentation and Evaluation

| 6. | A | 7. | D | 41. | C | 42. | A | 57. | A | 64. | B | 68. | D |
| 69. | C | 71. | A | 72. | A | 73. | D | 74. | B | 75. | C | 81. | C |

Organizing and Managing Services

| 32. | B | 33. | D | 39. | A | 60. | D | 70. | A | 80. | B | 87. | B |
| 88. | C |

Advancement of the Profession

| 9. | D | 65. | C | 79. | B | 89. | D | 90. | D |

Record Your Scores Here:

Background	____/ 7 =	____ %
Diagnostic Groupings	____/13 =	____ %
Assessment	____/14 =	____ %
Planning the Intervention	____/14 =	____ %
Implementing the Intervention	____/14 =	____ %
Documenting/Evaluation	____/14 =	____ %
Organizing/Managing	____/ 8 =	____ %
Advancement of the Profession	____/ 6 =	____ %

Total Score   ____/90

Total Percent   ____ %

If you need more practice in any area(s), proceed to Chapter Seven.

Chapter Seven
Diagnostic and Review Items

Before reaching this chapter, you have probably already completed the 270 items found in chapters five and six. These are intended to allow you to practice and score yourself on items similar to those found on the actual NCTRC exam.

The intent of this chapter is to provide a more in-depth practice experience that can be confined to your area(s) of weakness. You may complete all 240 items in this chapter or select only those categories in which you feel you need more help.

In chapter seven, there are 30 questions per each of the eight knowledge areas, for a total of 240 questions. Use these to help you determine if you do, in fact, need more study and preparation before taking the actual NCTRC exam.

If you find you need more information about a specific area, we advise you to return to chapter four, reread the information, and refer to the listing of resources given for each area. You may find that obtaining and reviewing a copy of these resources will be beneficial to you. You also may benefit from a study group of professional colleagues who can share resources and information. Regardless of how you help yourself prepare, make sure to leave enough time to become familiar with these areas before you take the test.

After additional study, you may want to retake the practice test or diagnostic items to see if you score better than the first time you tried. Try not to focus on these exact questions, but on the content which they represent. Always strive for a thorough understanding of the content, not just a quick memorization of the facts.

Diagnostic and Review Items

The sample questions that follow represent the types of questions included in the NCTRC Certification Exam. The purpose of these Diagnostic and Review Items is to give you some indication of the areas in which you may need additional preparation. The items are clustered by the eight knowledge areas.

Directions: For each question in this section, select the best of the answer choice given. Use the answer scoring sheet on page 179 to record your answers. Use the answer scoring key on page 180 to score your answers.

Background

1. Which of the following examples demonstrates the concept of "flow?"

    (A) Sharena got so involved in painting a sunset, she lost track of time.
    (B) Calvin, after trying a number of activities, decides he likes archery the best.
    (C) Katrina has three cats and two dogs and volunteers at the animal shelter twice a week.
    (D) Ian likes to travel to new places at least twice a year.

2. Which of the following example demonstrates the concept of "learned helplessness?"

    (A) Patricia plans on her calendar to do at least one fun thing per week.
    (B) Elizabeth has repeatedly failed and doesn't want to try any more.
    (C) Vanessa has trouble remembering to ask for help.
    (D) Douglas learned that asking for help is not a weakness.

3. Health can be defined, not just as the absence of illness, but as

    (A) a higher level of disease process
    (B) exercising three days a week for at least 30 minutes at a time
    (C) a sense of physical, mental, and social well-being
    (D) minimal deviation from normal functioning

4. The four basic measurable functions of health (blood pressure, pulse, respiration, and temperature) are called

    (A) vital signs
    (B) health signs
    (C) normal health signs
    (D) normal functioning

Questions 5-6

Using the following categories of child development, place the letter of the appropriate category in front of the skill that belongs in that category.

    I.   personal/social
    II. adaptive/fine motor behavior
    III. motor behavior
    IV. language

5. Takes turns

    (A) I only
    (B) II only
    (C) III only
    (D) IV only

6. Transfers cube from hand to hand

    (A) I only
    (B) II only
    (C) III only
    (D) IV only

7. In the continuum of therapeutic recreation services, the purpose of functional intervention services is to

    (A) provide cotreatment with other therapies at the most basic, functional levels
    (B) acquaint clients with available and appropriate community services
    (C) bring clients up to the baseline of their peers' average functional level
    (D) increase the physical capabilities of clients

8. According to the Leisure Ability model of therapeutic recreation services, the program service categories include

    (A) functional intervention, leisure education, and recreation participation services
    (B) therapy and recreation services
    (C) leisure education, counseling, and recreation services
    (D) inpatient, outpatient, and community services

9. In a facility that uses the Health Protection/Health Promotion model of therapeutic recreation, what would be the intent of service delivery?

    (A) Helping clients become more competent and able to select enjoyable activities
    (B) Helping people overcome barriers to health that interfere with their leisure
    (C) Promoting human happiness through primary and secondary efforts
    (D) Empowering the client to achieve only those goals that improve their leisure lifestyle

10. The "day-to-day behavioral expression of one's leisure-related attitudes, awareness, and activities revealed within the context and composite of the total life experience" is a person's

    (A) leisure lifestyle
    (B) recreation well being
    (C) quality of life
    (D) leisure well being

11. While a medical model of health focuses on the pathology of a person, the salutogenic model of health focuses on

   (A) lifestyle factors that support, enhance, and produce health
   (B) social relationships that need to be terminated prior to full recovery
   (C) total lifestyle environment to which the patient will return
   (D) direct reimbursement of services

Questions 12-13

Using the following Health Care Delivery Systems, select the one that most accurately reflects the statement given.

   I. Medical
   II. Custodial
   III. Milieu
   IV. Education and Training

12. This model is based on the philosophy that mental illness is the product of unhealthy interactions with one's environment.

   (A) I only
   (B) II only
   (C) III only
   (D) IV only

13. The primary therapist in this model is the professional who develops the most effective relationship with a particular client.

   (A) I only
   (B) II only
   (C) III only
   (D) IV only

14. In establishing an environment that embraces multiculturalism, the therapeutic recreation specialist would

   (A) make sure all ethnic holidays are on the activity calendar
   (B) introduce signage that includes both English and Spanish, and possibly French
   (C) recognize people's differences while establishing a sense of unity
   (D) follow the agency directives with regard to nondiscrimination toward foreigners

15. Which of the following statements about leisure's impact on coping with stressful life events is TRUE?

   (A) Leisure activities often intensify the harmful effects of negative life events.
   (B) Leisure activities often have the effect of eliminating optimism and hope about the future.
   (C) Leisure activities often disrupt one's ability to cope with stress.
   (D) Leisure activities may be used following negative life events to attain new goals.

16. The first step in a person changing a negative behavior to a positive behavior is

    (A) recognizing the problem behavior
    (B) reappraising the stressors that caused the original incident
    (C) coping with the negative consequences of the original behavior
    (D) believing the negative behavior can be changed.

17. The drug, Librium, is most often used to treat which of the following disorders?

    (A) Chronic angina
    (B) Anxiety
    (C) Muscle stiffness
    (D) Arrhythmias

18. Almost all models of therapeutic recreation service delivery start with the step of

    (A) assessment
    (B) goal development
    (C) program evaluation
    (D) quality improvement

19. In community-based therapeutic recreation programs, clients often self-select and preregister for   programs, which usually replaces the need for

    (A) assessment
    (B) program planning
    (C) leadership
    (D) a Certified Therapeutic Recreation Specialist

Questions 20-21

The most widely used therapeutic recreation service model consists of three areas of service provision. Select from the service provision areas listed above the one that BEST fits each of the following goal statements.

    I.   Functional Intervention
    II. Leisure Education
    III. Recreation Participation

20. To acquire problem-solving techniques for daily use

    (A) I only
    (B) II only
    (C) III only
    (D) I and II only

21. To encourage the client to focus on health and wellness rather than disease and pathology

    (A) I only
    (B) II only
    (C) III only
    (D) I and III only

22. Which of the following examples typify the theory of self-efficacy?

    (A) Josiah believes he is efficient in most leisure activities.
    (B) Colleen believes her life would change completely is she could live by herself.
    (C) Jacob hates to lose so tries extremely hard to excel so he can win.
    (D) Vijay believes he can master kayaking since he excels at canoeing.

23. The TRS provides many active games and sports to adolescents with emotional distur-bances to allow for the release of disorganized and pent-up emotions. The TRS adheres to which of the following theories of play?

    (A) Custodial
    (B) Psychoanalytical
    (C) Compensatory
    (D) Catharsis

24. During the 1960s and 1970s, society's view of health changed from one of "absence of illness" to the "state of complete physical, mental, and social well-being." How has this affected the provision of therapeutic recreation services?

    (A) They have become more segregated.
    (B) They have become less important to the treatment of individuals with health prob-lems.
    (C) They have been viewed as a preventative measure which helps alleviate health prob-lems.
    (D) They have not been affected.

25. Which of the following services was NOT mandated in the Community Mental Health Act of 1963?

    (A) Home health services
    (B) Inpatient hospitalization
    (C) Partial hospitalization
    (D) Community consultation and education

26. Inclusion is different than integration in what way?

    (A) Inclusion assumes the person has minimal disability to distract from the activity.
    (B) Inclusion only means a select group of higher functioning individuals.
    (C) Inclusion is required by federal, state, and local laws; integration is not.
    (D) Inclusion assumes the person has never been segregated.

27. Which of the following is an example of a self-fulfilling prophecy?

    (A) Hoosang enjoyed every minute of the self-awareness activity.
    (B) Susan felt great joy at helping other people, especially older adults.
    (C) Juan fails to make a point, just as his coach predicted.
    (D) Hillary always knew she wanted to be a therapeutic recreation specialist.

28. Ms. Brown has been admitted to a psychiatric facility for treatment of severe depression. The TRS suggests to her that she begin participating in a walking program and a peer communication program. She states to the TRS that she has never been able to walk very far, and has trouble communicating with others. She is not interested in the TR programs. Ms. Brown may be exhibiting

    (A) learned helplessness
    (B) infantile expressive skills
    (C) extrinsic behavior
    (D) aggressive behavior

29. The top two leading causes of death in the United States are

    (A) obesity and strokes
    (B) heart disease and cancers
    (C) heart disease and sexually-transmitted diseases
    (D) vehicular accidents and gun shot wounds

30. A person-centered approach to therapeutic recreation means that

    (A) despite differences, we accept that each individual is a unique person
    (B) we encourage age-appropriate behaviors and activities
    (C) we can reduce the impact of the self-fulfilling prophecy
    (D) we encourage clients to think of themselves first, others second

Diagnostic Groupings

1. An individual with a moderate hearing impairment would MOST likely need which of the following services or adaptations?

    (A) Community mobility training
    (B) Well-lit rooms with bright colors
    (C) Amplification devices in some situations
    (D) Personal assistants to take care of daily needs

2. Which of the following is an example of a secondary disability?

    (A) Osteoporosis and hip fracture
    (B) Spinal cord injury and heart disease
    (C) Dementia and losing track of time
    (D) Arthritis and scoliosis

3. Therapeutic recreation programs for individuals with acute schizophrenic disorders are MOST appropriate when they focus on goals to improve or increase

    (A) social interaction and motor behaviors
    (B) integration into community recreation activities
    (C) adaptive responses to addictive behaviors
    (D) manipulative behaviors of the client

4. The four axes of the Diagnostic and Statistical Manual IV-R are

    (A) physical, social, emotional, and intellectual disorders
    (B) clinical disorders, medical disorders, personality disorders, and psychosocial problems
    (C) anxiety disorders, affective disorders, substance abuse, and psychomotor disorders
    (D) schizophrenia, bi-polar disorder, substance abuse, and depression

5. Which of the following is the BEST example of a receptive communication dysfunction?

    (A) Inability to transform experiences into language
    (B) Inability to comprehend the written or spoken word
    (C) Inability to express oneself through actions or language
    (D) Inability to distinguish nuances in spoken language

6. Which of the following is NOT a symptom of substance use disorders?

    (A) Inability to distinguish healthy from non-healthy ways to cope with stress
    (B) Difficulty withdrawing or eliminating the substance from one's routine
    (C) Continued choice to use the substance despite problems associated with use
    (D) Change in the individuals' tolerance for the substance

7. Down syndrome, the best-known form of chromosomal mental retardation, is characterized by

    (A) short stature and enlarged rib cage and upper arms
    (B) flat, broad face and small ears and nose
    (C) increased urinary tract infections and sexual dysfunction
    (D) lowered IQ and osteoporosis

8. Feelings of overwhelming dread or impending doom with increased uneasiness are characteristics of

    (A) somatoform disorders
    (B) schizophrenia
    (C) anxiety disorders
    (D) multiple personality disorders

9.   Which of the following conditions is genetic, produces gradually wasting muscle, with accompanying weakness and deformity?

   (A) Spina bifida
   (B) Multiple sclerosis
   (C) Muscular dystrophy
   (D) Osteoarthritis

10. A client's symptoms of irritability, pallor, trembling, blurred vision, perspiration, fatigue, confusion and headache, may be indicators of

   (A) traumatic brain injury
   (B) diabetic coma
   (C) heart attack
   (D) post-traumatic stress syndrome

11. Alcohol is classified in which of the following categories of drugs?

   (A) Stimulants
   (B) Depressants
   (C) Hallucinogens
   (D) Narcotics

12. Alzheimer's type dementia is caused by

   (A) biological changes in the brain
   (B) getting older
   (C) not engaging in intellectual activities as one ages
   (D) environmental pollutants and toxins

13. The condition that exists when the effects of a drug have become necessary to the individual in order to maintain an optimal state of well-being, with an intensity ranging from mild desire to strong craving for the drug's effects is known as

   (A) drug abuse
   (B) psychological dependence
   (C) physical dependence
   (D) tolerance

14. People with depression often engage in _____ leisure activities, and report _____pleasure from participating.

   (A) more, more
   (B) more, less
   (C) fewer, more
   (D) fewer, less

15. One leadership principle the TRS should follow when working with autistic children is to

    (A) establish eye contact
    (B) use lengthy activities
    (C) play a lot of active games
    (D) change activities quickly

16. Which of the following activities has been proven to be most effective with improving psychological states?

    (A) soothing music
    (B) building bird houses
    (C) physical exercise
    (D) joining a social club

17. Neuroleptics is a class of medications used to treat

    (A) lower back pain
    (B) sociopathic disorders
    (C) epilepsy
    (D) schizophrenia

18. In human anatomy, the scapula performs what function?

    (A) It produces extensions and flexions of the upper leg.
    (B) It forms the shoulder joint where many bones and muscles originate.
    (C) It forms the elbow joint with the humerus proximally.
    (D) It serves as the foundation for speech.

19. To be classified as legally blind, a person must have visual acuity no better than

    (A) 20/20
    (B) 10/200
    (C) 20/200
    (D) 10/100

20. If an individual experiences a stroke on the right side of his/her brain, the typical effects include

    (A) lack of depth perception, intuition, and nonverbal perception
    (B) inability to remember past events and to read
    (C) inability to communicate and organize thoughts
    (D) increased lability and anger control

21. Typical treatment for a decubitus ulcer includes

    (A) increased cardiovascular exercise
    (B) a prescription for blood pressure medicine
    (C) bed rest and antibiotics
    (D) daily stress management classes

22. In the classical pattern of multiple sclerosis, the person experiences alternating intervals of

    (A) episodes of symptoms and remission
    (B) short mania and longer term depression
    (C) athetosis and ataxia
    (D) muscle atrophy and hypertonia

23. A TRS may work with a person who has recently experienced an extensive thermal burn, by providing which of the following types of services:

    (A) Communication techniques
    (B) Adjustment to disability sessions
    (C) Leisure awareness sessions
    (D) Assistive devices and adaptive techniques

24. Typical experiences of individuals with new spinal cord injuries include

    (A) heightened ability to cope with stress, fewer leisure options, and lowered self-esteem
    (B) decreased helplessness, fewer employment opportunities, and better relationships
    (C) loss of ability and skills, disruption of relationships, and dependence on others
    (D) higher risk for infections, lowered intellectual ability, and lowered self-esteem

Question 25

Consider the following statements about chronic pain.

    I.   Chronic pain is defined as pain that lasts more than six months.
    II. No major organic disorder can be found to explain chronic pain.
    III. The typical onset of chronic pain is the age of 41.
    IV. Chronic pain forms a cycle of lack of activity, then continued pain.

25. Which of the above represent true statements about chronic pain?

    (A) I only
    (B) I and II only
    (C) I, II and III only
    (D) I, II and IV only

26. Which of the following provides example behaviors from an individual with oppositional defiant behavior?

    (A) Extreme levels of hyperactivity and distractability
    (B) Interruptive social behaviors that are more apparent to others than the individual
    (C) Behaviors that violate the rights of others and major age-appropriate societal norms
    (D) Negative, hostile behaviors toward others

27. An individual who has a panic disorder experiences

    (A) maladaptive behaviors in response to social situations
    (B) persistent, abnormally intense fears
    (C) "free-floating" anxiety which tends to pervade all areas of life
    (D) sudden, periodic attacks of intense anxiety

28. Which of the following is a TRUE statement about autonomic hyperreflexia (Autonomic dysreflexia)?

    (A) It is often felt as an "aura" before the experience of a seizure.
    (B) Common in people with spinal cord injuries, it is a rapid and uncontrolled elevation in blood pressure.
    (C) It is common among individuals who have chronic schizophrenia and can be controlled through medication.
    (D) It is associated with excessive dopamine in the limbic brain center and eventually causes death.

29. Chronic users of cocaine may experience all of the following, EXCEPT:

    (A) Depression
    (B) Periods of excessive sleep
    (C) Hypertension
    (D) Respiratory and/or cardiac failure

30. Which of the following is a true statement about the aging process?

    (A) Individuals with less education tend to outlive those with more education
    (B) Women tend to outlive men
    (C) Ethnic minority members tend to outlive Caucasians
    (D) Individuals who are single tend to outlive those with families

Assessment

1. In order to place clients into a leisure education program, the TRS wants to assess social barriers to leisure involvement. Which of the following is the MOST appropriate content for the assessment instrument?

    (A) The ability to problem solve and make decisions
    (B) The ability to interact in group situations
    (C) The ability to control emotions
    (D) The ability to locate resources for leisure activities

2. What is likely to happen when the content of the assessment does not match the content of the programs designed for client participation?

    (A) The assessment is likely to be more valid than reliable.
    (B) The assessment will not lead to proper program placement and clients will not reach their goals.
    (C) Outcomes will be better defined and less ambiguous.
    (D) The assessment will have less cultural bias and increased sensitivity.

3. The purpose of an assessment protocol is to

   (A) make sure every client has the same diagnosis and treatment plan.
   (B) increase sensitivity to cultural minorities.
   (C) align the therapeutic recreation assessment with the occupational therapy assessment.
   (D) increase the reliability of the assessment administration.

4. If the client assessment cannot distinguish between those who need the program and those who do not, what is likely to happen to the clients?

   (A) They are likely to receive the wrong program, a diversional program, or no program at all.
   (B) They will receive both functional intervention and leisure education programs.
   (C) They are more likely to benefit from community integration programs.
   (D) They are more likely to efficiently reach their outcomes and achieve an early discharge.

5. The State Technical Institute's Leisure Assessment Process (STILAP) assessment differs from other activity inventories or leisure interest scales because it

   (A) focuses on physical activities such as sports and large group games
   (B) assesses barriers to community integration
   (C) looks at the entire community environment to which the client is to return
   (D) translates activity skills into leisure competencies

6. The purpose of client assessment is to

   (A) provide feedback on the effectiveness of an intervention program
   (B) place clients in programs based on their needs
   (C) improvement communication between members of the treatment team
   (D) evaluate client performance in therapeutic recreation programs

7. The overall content covered by the Leisure Diagnostic Battery (LDB) includes

   (A) leisure participation history
   (B) leisure interests
   (C) attitudes toward leisure and work
   (D) perceived freedom in leisure

8. Which of the following is most likely to produce error in a client's assessment score?

   (A) Lack of confidence in the therapeutic recreation specialist
   (B) Inconsistent administration of the assessment tool
   (C) Computerizing the assessment process
   (D) Following an assessment protocol

Questions 9-10

There are four basic types of observational recording systems. They include:

    I.   Frequency or Tallies
   II. Duration
  III. Interval
  IV. Continuous or Anecdotal

9.   Which of the following would be the most appropriate technique to record how many times a client uses negative self-statements?

   (A) I only
   (B) II only
   (C) I, II, and III only
   (D) I, II, III, and IV

10. Which of the following would be the most appropriate technique to record how long a client's anger outbursts last?

   (A) I only
   (B) II only
   (C) I, II, and III only
   (D) I, II, III, and IV

11. One method to increase inter-rater reliability in observations is to

   (A) improve the construct validity of the instrument
   (B) use clearly defined and non-overlapping categories
   (C) support the results with extensive interviews
   (D) purchase and compare similar interest inventories

12. If the client does not understand the language used on the assessment or becomes fatigued, what is likely to happen?

   (A) The therapeutic recreation specialist will gain insight into the sitting tolerance of the client.
   (B) The therapist still will be able to use the assessments from other disciplines to build a treatment plan.
   (C) Nothing, most therapeutic recreation specialists do not use assessment scores anyway.
   (D) The assessment score will not be reflective of the person's skills, attitudes, and knowledges.

13. A TRS selects the Comprehensive Evaluation in Recreational Therapy Scale (CERT) to measure behavior of a client as observed in group activities. Which assessment characteristic has the TRS considered in making this selection?

   (A) Validity
   (B) Reliability
   (C) Usability
   (D) Practicability

14. When an agency has decided to use the Functional Independence Measure (FIM), the TRS may be called upon to assess which of the following sections?

    (A) Self-care
    (B) Mobility
    (C) Communication
    (D) Social/cognition

15. When is it most appropriate to use structured observations for client assessment?

    (A) When actual behavior is of concern
    (B) When the person's perceptions of behaviors are important
    (C) When the person acts out in public
    (D) Rarely, interviews are always the better choice for client assessment purposes

16. Which of the following is an example of a probe that could be used during a client assessment?

    (A) My name is Reginald and I'd like to learn as much as I can today about your leisure.
    (B) To summarize your comments thus far....
    (C) And now let's move to the third section of the assessment.
    (D) Tell me more about your artistic ability.

17. A TRS is interested in determining a patient's leisure interests. From the following options, the TRS should choose which assessment?

    (A) Leisure Diagnostic Battery (LDB)
    (B) Leisurescope
    (C) Ohio Scales of Leisure Functioning
    (D) Comprehensive Evaluation in Recreational Therapy Scale (CERT)

18. A TRS is interested in determining behaviors that relate to a person's ability to successfully integrate into society using his/her social interaction skills. From the following options, the TRS should choose which assessment?

    (A) Leisure Diagnostic Battery (LDB)
    (B) Leisurescope
    (C) Ohio Scales of Leisure Functioning
    (D) Comprehensive Evaluation in Recreational Therapy Scale (CERT)

19. The TRS wants to make sure that the results of each client's assessment translates into the right program placement to work on the client's identified problems. What is the BEST method to make sure all TRs in the department translate client results in the same way?

    I.   Use an assessment that produces reliable scores for the intended population.
    II. Train all TRSs on the correct use of the assessment.
    III. Document a standardized protocol for the administration, scoring and interpretation of the assessment.
    IV. Improve the construct validity of the instrument.

(A) I and II only
(B) I, II, and III only
(C) II and III, only
(D) I, II, III, and IV

20. One of the major DISADVANTAGES of using interviews in client assessment is

(A) unless the scoring system is in place ahead of time, they are difficult to score and analyze.
(B) they are less likely to get correct information than observations.
(C) that clients often lie about their leisure participation patterns prior to admission.
(D) they reduce personal contact between the client and the therapeutic recreation specialist.

21. Which of the following is a question typical of a screening or intake assessment (vs. one that goes in more depth)?

(A) Does the client have adequate social skills?
(B) Does the client have adequate conversational skills with peers?
(C) If the client has difficulty conversing with peers, where does the difficulty lie?
(D) What difficulties have been improved or remedied by participation in the social skills program?

22. All of the following are examples of leisure barriers measured in the Leisure Barrier Inventory, EXCEPT:

(A) Time, money, and transportation
(B) Poor self-concept
(C) Availability of leisure partners
(D) Understanding of leisure as a concept

23. When an assessment is norm-referenced, it means that the assessment was/is

(A) interpreted based on the average scores for that person's peer group
(B) based on a normal population's average scores
(C) references using the major texts in the therapeutic recreation literature
(D) based on scores of normal behavior expected within that developmental life stage

Question 24

Consider the following two interview questions/statements to be used in a client assessment.
  A. "Tell me how you would go about finding transportation to get to an athletic event downtown."
  B. "Tell me about your family."

24. Interview question/statement A is better than B, because:

(A) It focuses on the specific content of therapeutic recreation programs.
(B) It requires less short-memory from the client.
(C) It requires less time for the client to answer.
(D) It takes more time to analyze and interpret the answer for placement into programs.

25. The Minimum Data Set (MDS) is an assessment completed for individuals in which type of setting?

    (A) Correctional institutions
    (B) Adult day care centers
    (C) Outpatient rehabilitation programs
    (D) Nursing homes

26. What effect has clients' shortened lengths of stay had on client assessment?

    (A) It is now a much easier task because clients are more focused on their own treatment.
    (B) The connection between gathering a baseline of information and measuring for outcomes has been strengthened.
    (C) Assessments need to be concise and administered more quickly following admission.
    (D) The effect has been minimal because therapeutic recreation specialists have always been known for efficient assessments.

27. One example of a "trigger" within the Activities section on the Minimum Data Set (MDS) would be when the individual

    (A) prefers more or different activity choices than are now being offered
    (B) rarely receives visits from family or friends
    (C) is completely independent in his/her leisure pursuits
    (D) is ready for discharge to his/her home

28. Unstructured interviews are usually less desirable than tests or directed observations to gather assessment data for which of the following reasons?

    I.   Individual TRSs may not use the same questions
    II. There is too much room for interpretation that limits reliability
    III. They are too difficult to score consistently

    (A) I only
    (B) I and II only
    (C) II and III only
    (D) I, II, and III

29. The TRS wants to assess clients for placement into a leisure education program. The TRS should make sure the instrument is valid and measures which of the following?

    (A) Social skills, leisure activity skills, leisure resources, and leisure awareness
    (B) Functional limitations, social skills, and physical abilities
    (C) Leisure interests, functional limitations, leisure awareness, and leisure resources
    (D) Decision-making skills, small group and large group interaction skills, and leisure resources

30. The results from any assessment should give the TRS a clear indication of

    (A) the programs in which the client should be placed
    (B) the client's leisure interests
    (C) the validity of the tool
    (D) how successful the client has been in achieving the program outcomes

Planning

1. A client outcome is the

    (A) client's heightened awareness of leisure as a substitute for work
    (B) observed changes in the client's status as a result of interventions
    (C) degree to which clients are satisfied with the treatment they have received
    (D) point at which activity analysis and client assessment intersect

2. In health care, the term capitation means the health care provider

    (A) agrees to a preset dollar amount per person and to not ask for further reimbursement
    (B) is reimbursed only for expenses that the client can pay for
    (C) must itemize all charges on the bill and relate each to a specific diagnosis code
    (D) is a member of a fee-for-service organization that agrees on charges prior to admission

3. Which of the following federal acts defined therapeutic recreation as a related area of service and was responsible for allowing more people with disabilities to be served by TRSs?

    (A) 1973 Rehabilitation Act
    (B) Smith-Sears Veterans Rehabilitation Act
    (C) Education of All Handicapped Children Act
    (D) White House Conference on Handicapped Individuals Act

4. Which of the following disciplines focuses on making and fitting hand braces?

    (A) Physical therapist
    (B) Nurses
    (C) Prosthetist
    (D) Orthotist

5. A clinical psychologist specializes in

    (A) diagnosing and treatment of mental illnesses
    (B) counseling victims of domestic violence
    (C) group therapy for a variety of psychoses
    (D) prescribing psychotropic drugs

Questions 6-8

    I. Condition
   II. Behavior
 III. Criteria

Written behavioral objectives that are measurable, contain the three major components listed above to specify what is expected from the patient/client. Examine each of the behavioral objectives listed below and determine whether each component is measurable. If a component is not measurable or missing, mark that letter. If the behavioral objective contains all three components, answer "D."

6.   Tonya will name four activities that she can do for free within her local community.

    (A) I only
    (B) II only
    (C) III only
    (D) It is written correctly.

7.   After completing the Stress Management program, Taneisha will name five effective methods for reducing daily stress.

    (A) I only
    (B) II only
    (C) III only
    (D) It is written correctly.

8.   When playing a board game, Alveda will wait his turn by:
    a. keeping his hands to himself;
    b. sitting quietly in his chair; and
    c. letting others take their appropriate turns, as judged by the therapeutic recreation specialist.

    (A) I only
    (B) II only
    (C) III only
    (D) It is written correctly.

9.   From assessment results, the TRS determines that Agatha has a lack of knowledge of community leisure facilities and programs, and is unaware of other people who participate in her leisure interests. Which of the following therapeutic recreation programs would be the MOST appropriate for this client?

    (A) Leisure planning
    (B) Social skills training
    (C) Leisure values and attitudes
    (D) Leisure resources

10. From assessment results, the TRS determines that Marshall has an inability to assert himself with peers or to follow through with commitments. He also lacks receptive communication skills. Which of the following therapeutic recreation programs would be MOST appropriate for this client?

    (A) Leisure planning
    (B) Social skills training
    (C) Leisure values and attitudes
    (D) Leisure resources

11. Programming that involves individual client assessment, individual program planning, implementation of a program, and evaluation of the effect of the program is often called

    (A) intervention programming
    (B) recreation for special populations
    (C) special recreation
    (D) activity programming

12. Inclusive recreation means that individuals with disabilities

    (A) attend segregated services before attending other programs
    (B) are mixed with individuals with dissimilar disabilities
    (C) are denied access to community programs because special programs are created
    (D) attend recreation programs of choice and have equal and joint participation

13. Which of the following is an example of a program based on the principle of "normalization?"

    (A) Older adults with sensory deficits are taken to a playground.
    (B) Female teenagers with developmental disabilities are taught music appreciation.
    (C) Youths in juvenile detention attend programs on vacationing overseas.
    (D) All children with disabilities are registered for community recreation programs.

14. When a hospital or health care agency receives accreditation from the Joint Commission on Accreditation of Healthcare Organizations, among other things, it means

    (A) the hospital will receive Medicare payments more easily
    (B) professionals working in the agency will get direct reimbursement for services
    (C) the client will receive a higher quality of care
    (D) client assessment must be completed with 12 hours of admission

15. Which of the following is an appropriate goal for a client who lacks awareness of personal resources?

    (A) The client will identify four assets within himself/herself that complement her leisure lifestyle.
    (B) The client will name three leisure resources in the community.
    (C) The client will learn three new leisure activities within the next three months.
    (D) The client will register for one community program within one month.

16. The therapist used a paper and pencil leisure education activity for a chronic mental health group. During the beginning of the activity, she realized that the clients could not read. The therapist did not adequately analyze the _____ requirements of the activity.

    (A) intellectual
    (B) affective
    (C) physical
    (D) administrative

17. Which of the following activity titles seem MOST appropriate to help clients develop social skills?

    (A) Bingo
    (B) Interaction skills for adults
    (C) Low-cost activities for children
    (D) Volleyball

18. Which of the following activity titles seem MOST appropriate to help clients develop skills to locate leisure resources in the community?

    (A) Low-cost activities for children
    (B) Activities that can be done at home
    (C) Using the telephone book
    (D) Creative expression for the future

19. Sara, a CTRS, knew that she could not program for and measure outcomes for self-esteem, but she still wanted to program in this area and have clients achieve measurable outcomes. What outcomes would be more appropriate than "improve self-esteem?"

    (A) Improve self-concept
    (B) Verbalize two positive statements about self
    (C) Decrease negative thoughts about self
    (D) Increase self-image

20. What has to be in alignment in order to produce measurable client outcomes?

    I.   Content of the assessment
    II. Goals written for the client
    III. Content of the program
    IV. Leisure education program

    (A) I and II only
    (B) I, II, and III only
    (C) I, II, III, and IV
    (D) none of the above

Questions 21-25

For the listed goal statements below, identify the behavioral area toward which intervention is directed.
- I. Cognitive
- II. Affective
- III. Physical
- IV. Social

21. To wait to interrupt until appropriate conversational opportunity occurs

    (A) I only
    (B) II only
    (C) III only
    (D) IV only

22. To ask for assistance when needed

    (A) I only
    (B) II only
    (C) III only
    (D) IV only

23. To improve ability to express anger in a positive manner

    (A) I only
    (B) II only
    (C) III only
    (D) IV only

24. To improve decision-making skills related to leisure involvement

    (A) I only
    (B) II only
    (C) III only
    (D) IV only

25. To increase standing tolerance to 15 minutes

    (A) I only
    (B) II only
    (C) III only
    (D) IV only

26. What is the primary focus of a systems approach to program planning?

    (A) Developing comprehensive agency strategic plans
    (B) Designing individual client implementation plans
    (C) Establishing protocols and evaluative standards
    (D) Determining the outcomes the program will accomplish

27. What is the relationship between goal statements and outcome measures?

    (A) Outcome measures are included in goal statements
    (B) Goals lead to the development of outcome measures
    (C) Goals are written for comprehensive program plans
    (D) Goals are for discharge plans and outcomes for treatment plans

28. Which of the following activities is MOST LIKELY to aid a client in increased physical endurance?

    (A) Leisure resource discussion group
    (B) Video games
    (C) Walking
    (D) Yoga

29. Considering the typical leisure patterns of adolescents, which activity choice is MOST LIKELY to be appropriate?

    (A) Community folk and social dance club
    (B) Square dancing
    (C) Building remote-controlled model airplanes
    (D) Crossword puzzles

30. Which of the following is of primary importance for the TRS to consider when selecting an intervention program that will produce a specific client outcome?

    (A) Resources necessary to offer the experiences
    (B) Staff skills needed to lead the activity
    (C) Functional requirements of the activity
    (D) Risk management protocols for the experience

Implementation

1. The therapeutic recreation specialist has clients discuss whether their daily behavior reflects their statements that their own personal health is of high importance. The specialist is using which of the following therapeutic recreation facilitation techniques?

    (A) Bibliotherapy
    (B) Remotivation
    (C) Resocialization
    (D) Values clarification

2. Biofeedback, meditation, autogenic training, and progressive muscle relaxation are examples of what kind of therapeutic recreation facilitation technique?

    (A) Relaxation training
    (B) Tai Chi
    (C) Guided imagery
    (D) Sensory stimulation

Questions 3-5

The TRS is leading a group of elderly, disoriented clients. She is using an intervention technique called Validation Therapy. This therapy has four phases. Using the program/interactions presented, decide which of the phases is being represented.

     I.   Birth of the Group—Creating Energy
    II.   Life of the Group—Verbal Interactions
  III.   Movement and Rhythms
  IV.   Closing of the Group with Anticipation for the Next Meeting

3.   Refreshments and an upbeat song

    (A) I only
    (B) II only
    (C) III only
    (D) IV only

4.   "Sometimes I feel very lonely and when I do, I go looking for a friend. Do you ever feel lonely, Mrs. Jones?"

    (A) I only
    (B) II only
    (C) III only
    (D) IV only

5.   "Mr. Smith did you remember to bring the poem you wanted to share with us? You did. Great! O.K., let's listen to Mr. Smith's poem."

    (A) I only
    (B) II only
    (C) III only
    (D) IV only

6.   A therapeutic recreation facilitation technique that focuses on taste, touch, sight, smell, hearing, and bodily movement, and is often combined with reminiscence and remotivation is called

    (A) sensory overload
    (B) aromatherapy
    (C) sensory stimulation
    (D) sensory integration

7.   All of the following assist individuals in coping with stress, EXCEPT their:

    (A) Attitudes of feeling challenged instead of threatened
    (B) Feelings of having adequate resources to deal with the situation
    (C) Type A personalities
    (D) Adequate social support networks

8. Stress management involves a variety of techniques, activities, and interventions designed to

   (A) reduce unfamiliar stress
   (B) cope more effectively with distress and add more positive stress (eustress)
   (C) increase the individual's capacity to take on and handle more stress
   (D) aid individuals who have recently suffered severe and significant losses

9. The TRS is teaching clients with panic disorders to breathe from their diaphragm, rather than their chest, because

   (A) diaphragmatic breathing exchanges a greater volume of air
   (B) diaphragmatic breathing can leave the individual light headed
   (C) chest breathing is harder to learn
   (D) the activity analysis showed that more people would be successful

10. Meditation is the practice of

    (A) resolving domestic violence conflicts
    (B) attempting to mindfully focus on one thought at a time
    (C) chanting mantras while in a yoga position
    (D) making clients responsible for their own behaviors

11. When he is upset or things do not go his way, Enrique lashes out at people, often making very caustic remarks and sometimes striking them. A therapeutic recreation facilitation technique that is MOST LIKELY to help Henry is called

    (A) journaling
    (B) reality therapy
    (C) resocialization
    (D) anger management

12. Which of the following is the BEST example of using visualization as a facilitation technique in therapeutic recreation?

    (A) Having a person with cancer imagine good cells chomping on cancerous cells
    (B) Asking a group to role play what they might do when a stranger approaches
    (C) Asking a group of clients to express their feelings through any visual art medium
    (D) Asking a client to paint a picture of her future leisure

13. Visualization can be helpful to clients because they can

    (A) use imaginary practice sessions for upcoming stressful situations
    (B) express their feelings without retribution from the group
    (C) relax at their own pace
    (D) only reveal to the group what they want to reveal

14. Biofeedback, as a stress management technique, can help individuals learn to modify all of the following bodily functions, EXCEPT:

    (A) Muscle tension
    (B) Skin surface temperature
    (C) Blood pressure
    (D) Rapid eye movement

15. Betsy tends to blame others when something goes wrong and has a difficult time accepting responsibility for her actions. What therapeutic recreation facilitation technique is MOST LIKELY to be helpful for Betsy?

    (A) Reality therapy
    (B) Anger management
    (C) Resocialization
    (D) Validation therapy

16. Why does "thought stopping" help reduce stress reactions in people who have obsessive or phobic thoughts?

    (A) Thoughts precede emotions which precede physiological responses.
    (B) It punishes them for their negative thoughts.
    (C) It isolates them from the group before they can be hurt.
    (D) It shows them they have value and worth.

17. Below are four steps of "thought stopping." In which order do the steps of thought stopping occur?

    I. Imagine the thought
    II. Thought substitution
    III. Aided thought interruption
    IV. Unaided thought interruption

    (A) I and III only
    (B) I, II and IV only
    (C) I, III, IV, and II
    (D) I, II, III, and IV

18. In Rational Emotive Therapy, the focus is placed on

    (A) irrational self-statements that interfere with a person's ability to see reality objectively
    (B) reducing stress by eliminating emotions that are not rational
    (C) paying attention to the physiological responses to stress
    (D) clarifying what the person thinks or feels about a situation

19. The therapeutic recreation specialist wants Sanchez to gain upper body strength so he can propel his wheelchair for longer distances. The TRS would MOST LIKELY use

    (A) stretching activities
    (B) wheelchair basketball
    (C) Tai Chi
    (D) anaerobic exercise

20. Time management is the practice of

    (A) structuring time to focus on important activities and minimizing unimportant activities
    (B) fitting more activities into a person's schedule
    (C) reducing the number of commitments on your time
    (D) keeping track of events and appointments in a personal calendar

21. People with chronic pain may benefit from time management sessions because

    (A) they tend to be the busiest people
    (B) they tend to be complainers and procrastinators
    (C) it would help them identify goals for spending their least painful time constructively
    (D) it would help them develop a beneficial exercise routine at a local community center

Questions 22-23

The following exchange took place between three clients, A, B, and C:

A: "I want you both to cover for me when the head nurse comes and asks why I wasn't in group therapy this morning."
B: "Okay, whatever you say."
C: "No, I can't do that for you, because that would be lying."

22. Client A was showing which of the following behavior styles?

    (A) Aggressive
    (B) Passive
    (C) Assertive
    (D) Emotive

23. Client C was showing which of the following behavior styles?

    (A) Aggressive
    (B) Passive
    (C) Assertive
    (D) Emotive

24. Which of the following concepts are premises of Reality Therapy?

    I. The specialist helps the client stay oriented to time, person and place.
    II. The client is responsible for all of his or her behavior.
    III. The specialist helps the client explore connections between past experiences and present actions.
    IV. The specialist helps the client focus on stopping irrational thoughts.

    (A) I only
    (B) II only
    (C) I, II, and III only
    (D) I, II, III, and IV

25. The client says that involvement with her family is very important to her, but spends an inordinate amount of time at work, usually bringing home a large pile of work to do in the evenings and on the weekends. The specialist may use what type of therapeutic technique to help her review her priorities and behaviors?

    (A) Values clarification
    (B) Reality orientation
    (C) Assertiveness training
    (D) Bibliotherapy

26. All of the following are examples of passive body language, EXCEPT:

    (A) Erect body posture
    (B) Apologetic tone of voice
    (C) Little eye contact
    (D) Hands kept in the lap

27. The TRS, in an assertiveness training session, teaches clients to avoid being persuaded by others into doing something against their wishes, by repeating a concise statement of refusal. The TRS is teaching clients the technique of

    (A) clouding
    (B) broken record
    (C) compromise
    (D) defusing

28. In order to benefit from aerobic exercise, individuals need to reach and stay within their target heart rate for at least twenty minutes. This formula for calculating target heart rate is

    (A) age minus 20, times 1.5
    (B) 60 to 75 percent of normal maximum heart rate
    (C) weight minus 15, plus age
    (D) 40 percent of normal maximum heart rate

29. The TRS brought a wedding album, rice, a bridal veil, and a ring pillow to the session to trigger older adults to talk about their past experiences about weddings. What technique was the TRS employing in this session?

    (A) Remotivation
    (B) Reality orientation
    (C) Reminiscing
    (D) Relaxation response

30. In order to teach adults appropriate social skills, the TRS task analyzes the skill of "beginning a conversation with a new person." All of the additional techniques would be appropriate to teach social skills, EXCEPT

    (A) demonstration by the TRS
    (B) practice and repetition by the client
    (C) practice with feedback from peers in the group
    (D) paper and pencil test

Documentation

1. Patient/client and program documentation are important because they allow which of the following?

    I. Increased communication among staff members
    II. A higher degree of accountability for services
    III. Information to be gathered to improve the total program

    (A) I and II only
    (B) I and II only
    (C) II and III only
    (D) I, II, and III

2. When the physician or treatment team creates a master list of patient/client deficits and develops a plan of action focused on these deficits, it is called which of the following?

    I. Problem-oriented medical records (POMR)
    II. Source-oriented medical records (SOMR)
    III. Quality improvement

    (A) I only
    (B) II only
    (C) II and III only
    (D) I, II, and III

3.   The therapeutic recreation specialist wrote the following note in a client's chart. Which of the following documentation principles was violated?

"Mrs. Sullivan appeared to be lethargic and depressed."

(A)   Be objective and factual in descriptions.
(B)   Be consistent and explain exceptional behavior.
(C)   Observe behavior, then write it down.
(D)   Focus on client behavior, rather than interpretations of behavior.

Question 4

The following is an excerpt from a patient's/client's treatment plan:

1.   Enroll pt. in Leisure Planning class Tuesdays and Thursdays. Focus on taking responsibility and decision-making.
2.   Enroll pt. in Social Singles Club weekly. Focus on initiating and maintaining conversations with peers.

4.   Which of the following, if any, was MOST likely identified as the patient's/client's problems?

(A)   A lack of knowledge of leisure resources and lack of social partners
(B)   A lack of conversational abilities and decreased concentration skills
(C)   A lack of repertoire of activity skills and inability to identify leisure value system
(D)   None of the above

Question 5

Compare the two progress notes written below:

(A)   Friday, 12/11 - Pt. seemed withdrawn on community outing Friday night.

(B)   Friday, 12/11 - While pt. was attending community outing Friday night, she conversed only once with other pts. for approximately one minute. Pt. remained alone in the corner of the van during transit, and stayed at a separate table during most of the night.

5.   Progress note B is the better written because it

(A)   states more consistent information
(B)   relies on professional judgments
(C)   states behavior rather than conclusions
(D)   uses less professional jargon

6.   All of the following may be questions that the therapeutic recreation specialist uses to improve clarity and completeness to a narrative note EXCEPT:

(A)   How did I first become aware of the problem?
(B)   What has the client said about the problem that is not significant?
(C)   Is this the same problem that was exhibited last week?
(D)   What is the plan for dealing with the problem?

7. In problem-oriented record keeping, the abbreviation SOAPIER stands for

   (A) Subjectivity, Objectivity, Assess, Plan, Implement, Evaluate, Revise
   (B) Subjective data, Objective data, Analysis, Plan, Interventions, Evaluation, Revisions
   (C) Sources, Objects, Adjectives, Protocols, Initiatives, Expressions, Resolutions
   (D) nothing, it simply means to completely cover (saturate) the topic

8. In order for charting-by-exception to be effective, what first must be accomplished?

   (A) Standards of care must be predefined so exceptions can be identified.
   (B) The patient must be medically stable and coherent.
   (C) Reimbursement for services has to be standardized hospital-wide.
   (D) All health care professions must agree to a single page assessment form.

9. What is an advantage of asking open-ended questions of clients for a program evaluation?

   (A) The answers are easily quantifiable.
   (B) The clients are able to expand on their answers.
   (C) The specialist needs to be skilled in interviewing people.
   (D) There is no advantage to open-ended questions.

10. Which of the following would NOT be a problem-strength area used for client documentation by therapeutic recreation specialists?

    (A) Physical, emotional, and leisure functioning
    (B) Social/personal functioning, psychological functioning, and leisure interests
    (C) Self-esteem, activities of daily living, and leisure history
    (D) Independent living skills, social/personal functioning, and leisure functioning

11. The specialist tracks the number of times a client responds appropriately to another peer, in order to monitor the effects of the social skills program. This type of observation is being recorded through the _____ method.

    (A) tally
    (B) duration
    (C) interval
    (D) instantaneous time sampling

12. The program evaluation is designed at the same time the program is planned so that the

    (A) specialist will know how and when to collect information as the program progresses
    (B) client will know from the activity calendar when activities are offered
    (C) treatment team can collect information about the continuity of care
    (D) activities are analyzed for their physical, social/affective, and intellectual requirements of clients

13. Which question is a formative evaluation concern?

    (A) How does the second day of the program need to be changed from the first day?
    (B) Are the interventions appropriate for the content?
    (C) What were the total resource costs of program delivery
    (D) Were staff adequately prepared to deliver the services to this group of clients?

Questions 14-17

Using the following documentation sample, identify the abbreviation/symbol with the correct word or words.

Pt. is a 73 yo ♀ s/p Rt CVA c̄ Lt. hemiparesis. Oriented x3. MS intact. PMH significant for CAD, IDDM. Encourage Pt. up ad. lib. Appears to be dependent w/c. PT consult for ambulating, OT consult for ADL, TR consult for community reintegration.

14. Pt. is the abbreviation for
    (A) patient
    (B) physical therapy
    (C) private
    (D) point of concern

15. "yo" is the abbreviation for

    (A) hello
    (B) year old
    (C) youthful appearing
    (D) young at heart

16. Rt is the abbreviation for

    (A) recreation therapy
    (B) reality therapy
    (C) remotivation therapy
    (D) right

17. c̄ is the abbreviation for

    (A) cover
    (B) with
    (C) under
    (D) about

18. Which of the following is an example of the condition part of a behavioral objective?

    (A) With level 4 minimal assistance
    (B) The client will plan a weekend trip
    (C) Within ten minutes
    (D) Two out of three times

19. Which of the following questions would NOT be appropriate when documenting a client's participation in a therapeutic recreation program?

    (A) Did the client attend voluntarily?
    (B) Did the client merely observe the activity?
    (C) Was the client actively participating in the session?
    (D) Did the client attend all of the programs on Tuesday?

20. The therapeutic recreation specialist may need to describe specific behavioral cues that help describe the client's behavior. The client's _____ can be described using words such as lively, neutral, blunted, flat, stable, labile, defensive, calm, sad, hostile, guarded, distant, evasive, cooperative, and open.

    (A) speech
    (B) mood and effect
    (C) social distancing
    (D) movement

21. Kiki and Devon ran away during a community outing. After contacting the police, the therapeutic recreation specialist completes what form?

    (A) Incident report
    (B) Revised treatment plan
    (C) Discharge/referral summary
    (D) Liability summary

22. The basic premise behind "managed care" in the health care industry is

    (A) positive client outcomes produced at low cost
    (B) less focus on the individual, more focus on the diagnosis
    (C) sustaining a person's life at all costs
    (D) that insurance companies will pay whatever the clinical facilty charges for a service

23. One document within a written plan of operation is the department's or unit's scope of care. The scope of care specifies

    (A) the comprehensive goals and program areas of the department
    (B) methods of treating groups of clients
    (C) the treatment protocols for specific diagnostic groups
    (D) how the TRS should interact with the clients

24. All of the following areas of a TR department's written plan of operation may have specific, written policies and procedures, EXCEPT:

    (A) Obtaining physician's orders for treatment of clients
    (B) Employee hiring and firing procedures
    (C) How TRSs apply for recertification
    (D) Procedures for obtaining supplies from the dietary department

25. In calculating the price to be charged the client in a fee-for-service arrangement, the TRS should consider which of the following costs?

    (A) Direct costs, indirect costs, and uncollectibles (individuals unable to pay)
    (B) Department budget, divided by the number of therapeutic recreation programs
    (C) Department budget, divided by the number of therapeutic recreation staff
    (D) Staff salaries, facility rental, and overhead costs

26. Which of the following documents help support direct reimbursement for TR services?

    (A) Client assessment, treatment protocols, and quality improvement documents
    (B) Flow charts and trend analysis
    (C) Utilization review documents, treatment protocols, and risk management studies
    (D) Policy and procedures manuals

27. Which of the following might be an outcome indicator assessed through a continuous quality improvement program?

    (A) Qualifications of the TR staff
    (B) Environment in which treatment is provided
    (C) Intervention strategies employed by the TRS
    (D) Changes in the client's functional capacity

28. Which of the following is not an example of a TR department's risk management plan?

    (A) Requiring TR student interns to purchase liability insurance before the internship starts
    (B) Requiring employees to park on hospital premises
    (C) Conducting peer reviews by trained professionals
    (D) Incorporating family into the assessment procedure

29. The TR department director is instructed to prepare a zero-based budget for the upcoming fiscal year. This means that the TR director

    (A) adds a certain percentage to last year's budget to calculate this year's budget
    (B) receives no salary raise for the upcoming year
    (C) builds this year's budget from scratch
    (D) must negotiate with other departments to get more money in the budget

30. All of the following may be part of the department's risk management plan, EXCEPT:

    (A) Acceptable staff/client ratios for certain types of programs
    (B) Qualifications and special certifications needed by staff
    (C) Marketing brochures for fund raising purposes
    (D) Procedures for reporting emergencies, crises, and critical incidents

Organizing

1. The Centers for Medicare and Medicaid Services (CMS, formerly the Health Care Financing Administration [HCFA]) monitors quality assessment and performance improvement in facilities that

    (A) serve individuals covered by the federal government's health insurance program.
    (B) use the Therapeutic Recreation Accountability Model.
    (C) adhere to the National Therapeutic Recreation Society's Standards of Practice.
    (D) are located in low-income, urban areas.

2. Which of the following statements reflect the current emphasis of external accreditation agencies in reviewing therapeutic recreation services for quality improvement purposes?

    (A) The effectiveness of therapeutic recreation services is determined by the achieved client outcomes.
    (B) The most important criteria for proving effectiveness of therapeutic recreation services is the availability of facilities and adequacy of equipment.
    (C) The crucial element in therapeutic recreation quality assurance is the interaction established between the TRS and the client.
    (D) Linkages with community agencies is the prime factor in determining quality care in therapeutic recreation services.

Questions 3-5

Refer to the following excerpt from a sample quality improvement documentation.

Major Aspect of Care: Community Leisure Involvement Post-Discharge
Indicator: Increase in independent involvement in community recreation activities and opportunities
Criterion: Average of two community involvements per month following discharge per 80% of the clients
Standard: Review 10 percent of client follow-up forms
Data Source: Follow-up Client Interview Form

3. Which of the following components represents the therapeutic recreation department's definition of important or crucial elements of the therapeutic recreation service?

    (A) Major aspect of care
    (B) Indicator
    (C) Criterion
    (D) Standard

4. The documentation above is based upon which of the following focuses, if any?

    (A) Structure
    (B) Process
    (C) Outcomes
    (D) None

5. The therapeutic recreation department would determine if it was providing quality care by

   (A) completing program evaluations with clients at the end of 10% of the programs
   (B) finding that 10% of all clients reviewed averaged at least two community involvements per month
   (C) measuring the total number of client community involvements and dividing by 10
   (D) referring 10% of the clients to community-based therapeutic recreation programs post-discharge

Question 6

Which of the following show the order of the steps involved in creating a job description for a new position for a Therapeutic Recreation Specialist?

   I. Review NCTRC Job Analysis Study for entry-level competencies
   II. Identify the important job tasks of the vacant or new position
   III. Create a vision statement for the job position
   IV. Identify the qualifications that fit the job tasks of the position
   V. Check with the Human Resources department of the organization

6. (A) I, II, III, IV, V
   (B) I, II, IV
   (C) V, I, II, IV
   (D) IV, II, V, I, II

7. An advantage of calling someone's references before hiring him is that the supervisor can

   (A) ask the reference to compare qualifications of several applicants
   (B) ask about personal issues such as family status, drug and alcohol history, and religion
   (C) verify information from the resume or interview
   (D) orient the employee to hospital procedures and introduce staff of different departments

8. Which of the examples below illustrates using the principles of evidence-based research in therapeutic recreation?

   (A) The therapeutic recreation specialist uses results from a *Therapeutic Recreation Journal* article to most efficiently create a stress management program.
   (B) The therapeutic recreation specialist collects evidence over 12 months to show the attendance rates of clients.
   (C) The therapeutic recreation specialist attends a research forum at a national conference.
   (D) The therapeutic recreation specialist calls colleagues to see how their aquatic programs are designed.

9. Facilities that provide adult day care, assisted living, behavioral health, and employment and community services are MOST LIKELY to seek accreditation from

   (A) Joint Commission on Accreditation of Healthcare Organizations (JCAHO)
   (B) National Committee for Quality Assurance (NCQA)
   (C) Centers for Medicare and Medicaid Services (CMS)
   (D) Rehabilitation Accreditation Commission (CARF)

10. Which of the following may be used as a technique to motivate employees on a long-term basis?

    (A) Make them boss for the day
    (B) Set long- and short-term goals for them
    (C) Encourage their donations to the agency's charity fund
    (D) Encourage cross training into new areas of job responsibility

Questions 11-12

Natalissa is the supervisor of a large therapeutic recreation department in a community mental health center. The department has 12 therapeutic recreation staff, six of who are NCTRC certified. The staff is split evenly between an adult unit and an adolescent unit. When staff cutbacks were ordered in the TR department by the center's administrators, she ignored the memos and continued to staff the units on regular schedules.

11. The conflict resolution strategy employed by Natalissa is called _____ .

    (A) avoidance
    (B) defusion
    (C) containment
    (D) confrontation

12. Had she employed a strategy that involved problem-solving and direct conversations with the administrators, she would have been using the _____ strategy of conflict resolution.

    (A) avoidance
    (B) defusion
    (C) containment
    (D) confrontation

13. A TRS was hired to create a new department from "scratch," and will be hiring new personnel, determining the nature and direction of programs, and supervising the overall operation of the department. Which of the following resources would be MOST appropriate to review prior to creating this department?

    (A) *Guidelines for Administration of Therapeutic Recreation Services in Clinical and Residential Facilities* (NTRS)
    (B) *Code of Ethics* (ATRA)
    (C) *Therapeutic Recreation Journal* (NTRS)
    (D) *Evaluation of Therapeutic Recreation Through Quality Assurance* (ATRA)

14. Which of the following is a team-building strategy for personnel within a therapeutic recreation department?

    (A) Establish goals that are to be accomplished as a group
    (B) Implement policies without staff input
    (C) Keep the information flow to a minimum
    (D) Make unilateral decisions

15. Which of the following is NOT a characteristic of "high performance teams" of people working in a health care environment?

    (A) Decisions are made by group members
    (B) Each person shares in the responsibility for success
    (C) Each person is responsible for someone else's job
    (D) Responses to requests are timely and efficient

16. Knowing the payer mix of the agency is important because it

    (A) influences how external accreditation agencies review the various departments
    (B) requires an extensive knowledge of insurance company forms
    (C) influences how the agency gets reimbursed for services
    (D) shortens the patient's length of stay

17. Managed care is an effort on behalf of insurance companies to

    (A) increase patient's length of stay
    (B) control costs of caring for clients
    (C) reduce the paperwork involved in client care
    (D) decrease the number of preferred provider organizations (PPOs)

18. A strategic plan is a method of

    (A) projecting needs and activities of an organization in the future
    (B) continuous quality improvement
    (C) protocol development and implementation
    (D) resource utilization

19. The difference between a vision statement and a statement of purpose for an organization is that a vision statement is

    (A) never put into operation
    (B) created solely by the top level managers
    (C) far-reaching and translates values into a desired future
    (D) is for the immediate future and is directly translated into operational goals

20. The difference between an operational budget and a capital budget is that an operational budget

    (A) includes large expenditures of any kind over $500
    (B) covers all revenues and expenditures, except personnel
    (C) covers day-to-day revenues and expenditures for a one-year period
    (D) has line-items that can be vetoed by the agency president

21. A marketing audit is a vital step in designing a marketing plan for a therapeutic recreation department because it

    (A) describes what past marketing efforts and effects have been
    (B) evaluates the target audiences and the information they seek
    (C) critiques what others have done in the area
    (D) establishs goals and objectives for implementation

22. For a service to be reimbursable, in many instances insurance companies require the therapist to provide what information or evidence?

    (A) Assessment tools sanctioned by JCAHO, HCFA, or CARF
    (B) Source-oriented medical records
    (C) Physicians orders
    (D) Risk management plan for the activity

23. A clinical TR specialist and a community TR specialist are conducting a marketing analysis to set-up a joint out-patient rehab program. Which statement identifies a factor that would be considered an opportunity to promote this joint venture?

    (A) PT and OT are currently contracting their services in the community
    (B) A private health care company is providing in-home care in the area
    (C) Patient length of stay in inpatient rehabilitation is continuing to decrease
    (D) An ADA survey is presently being conducted in the community

24. Which organization oversees the accreditation of rehabilitation facilities?

    (A) Joint Commission of Accreditation of Healthcare Organizations (JCAHO)
    (B) Rehabilitation Accreditation Commission (CARF)
    (C) American Therapeutic Recreation Association (ATRA)
    (D) Centers for Medicare and Medicaid Services (CMS)

25. The Joint Commission identifies three categories of outcome measures: health status, patient perceptions of care, and client performance outcomes. The therapeutic recreation specialist reports on leisure interests, which falls in which of the following outcome categories?

    (A) Health status
    (B) Patient perceptions of care
    (C) Client performance outcomes
    (D) None of the above

26. Managed care has shifted the responsibility of determining the services a patient need from the _____ to the _____.

    (A) federal government, state governments
    (B) providers of service, payers of service
    (C) patient, insurance company
    (D) upper class, middle class

27. In a prospective payment system of health care, the hospital knows that a specific amount will be paid by the insurance company for a particular surgery, regardless of the _____.

    (A) skill of the surgeon
    (B) ethnicity of the patient
    (C) actual cost of the surgery
    (D) intended outcomes

28. In a therapeutic recreation program accredited by JCAHO, which phrase would the TRS be more likely to include in the department's mission statement?

    (A) The intent of services is to enhance client capacity to function independently in life activities.
    (B) The focus of intervention is on the removal of leisure barriers.
    (C) Clients participate in therapeutic recreation to enhance leisure awareness.
    (D) Services are monitored to ensure improvement in problem solving.

29. A patient was discharged from the clinical facility because it was determined that he was not making progress and the bed space was needed for incoming patients. Which of the following committees/departments would make this type of decision?

    (A) Professional standards review organization
    (B) Utilization review
    (C) Medical records review
    (C) Quality improvement

30. Which of the following is NOT appropriate in the therapeutic recreation department's written plan of operation?

    (A) The mission, vision, and goals of the unit
    (B) Comprehensive and specific program protocols
    (C) The listing of assessments, evaluation, and their administrative procedures
    (D) Individual clients' treatment and program plans

Advancement of the Profession

1. A TRS working in a psychiatric facility needs to find information about specific mental illnesses and conditions. Which of the following references would be MOST appropriate?

    (A) Physicians' Desk Reference
    (B) Diagnostic and Statistical Manual–IV
    (C) Therapeutic Recreation and the Nature of Disabilities (Mobily & MacNeil)
    (D) Comprehensive Accreditation Manual for Behavioral Health Care (JCAHO)

2. The most recent and the most preferred national standards for accessibility are contained within the

    (A) Joint Commission on Accreditation of Healthcare Organization's standards manuals
    (B) Accessibility Guidelines for America
    (C) Department of the Interior's park and natural areas guidelines
    (D) Americans with Disabilities Act

3. The intent of the federal initiative called Healthy People 2010 is to

    (A) heighten awareness of the overall health of Americans, including those with disabilities
    (B) ensure that Americans understand that eating fast food is the prime predictor of obesity
    (C) monitor the increasing amount of time Americans are spending on exercising
    (D) monitor the effects of low-carbohydrate diets on the obesity of Americans

4. It is the responsibility of every TRS to advocate for the leisure rights of individuals with disabilities because it is a(n)

    (A) privilege
    (B) option
    (C) right
    (D) challenge

5. Which of the following statements is NOT a suggested principle for structuring inclusionary programs?

    (A) Exempt the person with the disability from rules that require physical or intellectual skill.
    (B) Rotate positions and roles of the participants within the activity or program.
    (C) Role model positive, accepting behavior as the leader of the activity or program.
    (D) Accent positive attributes and skills of all participants.

6. The organization that provide personnel standards for therapeutic recreation specialists is

    (A) National Therapeutic Recreation Society (NTRS)
    (B) American Therapeutic Recreation Association (ATRA)
    (C) National Council for Therapeutic Recreation Certification (NCTRC)
    (D) Joint Commission of Accreditation of Healthcare Organizations (JCAHO)

7. What piece of legislation mandated program accessibility?

    (A) Americans with Disabilities Act of 1990
    (B) Section 504 of the 1973 Vocational Rehabilitation Amendments
    (C) Architectural Barriers Act of 1968
    (D) Public Law 94-142 of 1975

8. Approximately what percentage of Therapeutic Recreation Specialists are employed in community- based settings?

    (A) About 5 percent
    (B) About 15 percent
    (C) About 25 percent
    (D) About 35 percent

9. The purpose of accreditation of higher education programs for therapeutic recreation is to

    (A) guarantee that graduates are automatically certified by NCTRC
    (B) ensure compliance with NTRS and ATRA standards of practice
    (C) ensure that the programs meet national standards for the preparation of professionals
    (D) verify that faculty are certified by NCTRC

10. Which of the following is NOT a method for a CTRS to be recertified by NCTRC?

    (A) Receiving a passing grade in university-level course work
    (B) Completing a second internship in a different setting
    (C) Attending professional workshops that award CEUs for participation
    (D) Writing and publishing educational articles in professional journals

11. The process by which an agency or organization evaluates and recognizes a program of study or an institution as meeting certain predetermined qualifications or standards is called _____ .

    (A) licensure
    (B) accreditation
    (C) certification
    (D) registration

12. A TRS should use which of the following resources to find successful, proven methods of achieving positive client outcomes through actual therapeutic recreation services?

    (A) *Therapeutic Recreation Journal*
    (B) An introduction to therapeutic recreation textbook
    (C) *Adapted Activities Quarterly*
    (D) A therapeutic recreation programming textbook

13. The process by which an agency of the government grants permission to persons meeting predetermined qualification to engage in a given occupation is called _____ .

    (A) licensure
    (B) accreditation
    (C) certification
    (D) registration

14. The process by which qualified individuals are listed on an official roster maintained by a governmental or non-governmental agency is called _____ .

    (A) licensure
    (B) accreditation
    (C) certification
    (D) registration

15. Educating others about a particular issue is called

    (A) education for all
    (B) advocacy
    (C) wellness promotion
    (D) attitude adjustment

Questions 16-19

Using the following examples, determine which principle from the ATRA Code of Ethics is being represented.

    I.   Principle 2: Autonomy
    II. Principle 3: Veracity/Informed Consent
    III. Principle 4: Competence
    IV. Principle 7: Confidentiality and Privacy

16. The TRS works with an educator from a local university to research the impact of exercise on substance abuse patients in an outpatient recovery program.

    (A) I
    (B) II
    (C) III
    (D) IV

17. The TRS is treating a divorced parent who has custody of two children. The lawyer of the non-custodial parent calls seeking information regarding the status of the parent. The TRS refuses to give information.

    (A) I
    (B) II
    (C) III
    (D) IV

18. Patients have the right to have the treatment plan explained to them.

    (A) I
    (B) II
    (C) III
    (D) IV

19. The TRS sends in forms reporting participation in continuing education activities to NCTRC every five years.

    (A) I
    (B) II
    (C) III
    (D) IV

20. ATRA's *Standards for the Practice of Therapeutic Recreation* document is divided into two sections of

    (A) assessment and program planning
    (B) clinical and community guidelines
    (C) direct practice and management
    (D) inpatient and outpatient care

21. ATRA's fifth *Standard of Practice* relates to

    (A) recreation services
    (B) assessment
    (C) evaluation
    (D) discharge planning

22. ATRA's first *Standard of Practice* relates to

    (A) treatment planning
    (B) assessment
    (C) evaluation
    (D) ethical conduct

23. One of the principles in ATRA's *Code of Ethics* is Beneficience/Nonmalfeasance. This concept means

    (A) all individuals should receive identical services
    (B) all client have the basic right of self-determination
    (C) at best, provide benefit; at worst, do no harm
    (D) that confidentiality is expected in almost all situations

24. One of the principles in ATRA's *Code of Ethics* is Veracity/Informed Consent. This concept means

    (A) all client data must be verified by a third party prior to any treatment
    (B) insurance companies have the right to limit the amount of payment for any service
    (C) clients have the right to know the benefits and risks prior to participation
    (D) clients' photographs cannot be taken with their permission

25. The NTRS's *Code of Ethics* addresses its ethical standards in relation to

    (A) requirements
    (B) needs
    (C) obligations
    (D) essentials

26. The organization that is responsible for the certification of TR professionals is called
    _____ .

    (A) ATRA
    (B) NTRS
    (C) NRPA
    (D) NCTRC

27. What group is responsible for the accreditation of TR educational programs in universities and colleges?

    (A) JCAHO
    (B) CARF
    (C) COA
    (D) NCTRC

28. What professional organization was formed by the merger of several organizations?

    (A) NCTRC
    (B) NTRS
    (C) ATRA
    (D) CARF

29. What professional organization was formed out of the need to have a professional organization that could more easily respond to the clinical needs of the profession?

    (A) NCTRC
    (B) NTRS
    (C) ATRA
    (D) CARF

30. Networking is helpful to therapeutic recreation specialists because

    (A) expertise and ideas are shared to improve the quality of programs
    (B) each professional can claim a unique set of skills
    (C) clients are not likely to know more than one therapeutic recreation specialist
    (D) individuals with disabilities are likely to receive fewer services in the future

Diagnostic and Review Items
Answer Scoring Sheet

Background

1. Ⓐ Ⓑ Ⓒ Ⓓ	11. Ⓐ Ⓑ Ⓒ Ⓓ	21. Ⓐ Ⓑ Ⓒ Ⓓ
2. Ⓐ Ⓑ Ⓒ Ⓓ	12. Ⓐ Ⓑ Ⓒ Ⓓ	22. Ⓐ Ⓑ Ⓒ Ⓓ
3. Ⓐ Ⓑ Ⓒ Ⓓ	13. Ⓐ Ⓑ Ⓒ Ⓓ	23. Ⓐ Ⓑ Ⓒ Ⓓ
4. Ⓐ Ⓑ Ⓒ Ⓓ	14. Ⓐ Ⓑ Ⓒ Ⓓ	24. Ⓐ Ⓑ Ⓒ Ⓓ
5. Ⓐ Ⓑ Ⓒ Ⓓ	15. Ⓐ Ⓑ Ⓒ Ⓓ	25. Ⓐ Ⓑ Ⓒ Ⓓ
6. Ⓐ Ⓑ Ⓒ Ⓓ	16. Ⓐ Ⓑ Ⓒ Ⓓ	26. Ⓐ Ⓑ Ⓒ Ⓓ
7. Ⓐ Ⓑ Ⓒ Ⓓ	17. Ⓐ Ⓑ Ⓒ Ⓓ	27. Ⓐ Ⓑ Ⓒ Ⓓ
8. Ⓐ Ⓑ Ⓒ Ⓓ	18. Ⓐ Ⓑ Ⓒ Ⓓ	28. Ⓐ Ⓑ Ⓒ Ⓓ
9. Ⓐ Ⓑ Ⓒ Ⓓ	19. Ⓐ Ⓑ Ⓒ Ⓓ	29. Ⓐ Ⓑ Ⓒ Ⓓ
10. Ⓐ Ⓑ Ⓒ Ⓓ	20. Ⓐ Ⓑ Ⓒ Ⓓ	30. Ⓐ Ⓑ Ⓒ Ⓓ

Diagnostic Groupings

1. Ⓐ Ⓑ Ⓒ Ⓓ	11. Ⓐ Ⓑ Ⓒ Ⓓ	21. Ⓐ Ⓑ Ⓒ Ⓓ
2. Ⓐ Ⓑ Ⓒ Ⓓ	12. Ⓐ Ⓑ Ⓒ Ⓓ	22. Ⓐ Ⓑ Ⓒ Ⓓ
3. Ⓐ Ⓑ Ⓒ Ⓓ	13. Ⓐ Ⓑ Ⓒ Ⓓ	23. Ⓐ Ⓑ Ⓒ Ⓓ
4. Ⓐ Ⓑ Ⓒ Ⓓ	14. Ⓐ Ⓑ Ⓒ Ⓓ	24. Ⓐ Ⓑ Ⓒ Ⓓ
5. Ⓐ Ⓑ Ⓒ Ⓓ	15. Ⓐ Ⓑ Ⓒ Ⓓ	25. Ⓐ Ⓑ Ⓒ Ⓓ
6. Ⓐ Ⓑ Ⓒ Ⓓ	16. Ⓐ Ⓑ Ⓒ Ⓓ	26. Ⓐ Ⓑ Ⓒ Ⓓ
7. Ⓐ Ⓑ Ⓒ Ⓓ	17. Ⓐ Ⓑ Ⓒ Ⓓ	27. Ⓐ Ⓑ Ⓒ Ⓓ
8. Ⓐ Ⓑ Ⓒ Ⓓ	18. Ⓐ Ⓑ Ⓒ Ⓓ	28. Ⓐ Ⓑ Ⓒ Ⓓ
9. Ⓐ Ⓑ Ⓒ Ⓓ	19. Ⓐ Ⓑ Ⓒ Ⓓ	29. Ⓐ Ⓑ Ⓒ Ⓓ
10. Ⓐ Ⓑ Ⓒ Ⓓ	20. Ⓐ Ⓑ Ⓒ Ⓓ	30. Ⓐ Ⓑ Ⓒ Ⓓ

Assessment

1. Ⓐ Ⓑ Ⓒ Ⓓ	11. Ⓐ Ⓑ Ⓒ Ⓓ	21. Ⓐ Ⓑ Ⓒ Ⓓ
2. Ⓐ Ⓑ Ⓒ Ⓓ	12. Ⓐ Ⓑ Ⓒ Ⓓ	22. Ⓐ Ⓑ Ⓒ Ⓓ
3. Ⓐ Ⓑ Ⓒ Ⓓ	13. Ⓐ Ⓑ Ⓒ Ⓓ	23. Ⓐ Ⓑ Ⓒ Ⓓ
4. Ⓐ Ⓑ Ⓒ Ⓓ	14. Ⓐ Ⓑ Ⓒ Ⓓ	24. Ⓐ Ⓑ Ⓒ Ⓓ
5. Ⓐ Ⓑ Ⓒ Ⓓ	15. Ⓐ Ⓑ Ⓒ Ⓓ	25. Ⓐ Ⓑ Ⓒ Ⓓ
6. Ⓐ Ⓑ Ⓒ Ⓓ	16. Ⓐ Ⓑ Ⓒ Ⓓ	26. Ⓐ Ⓑ Ⓒ Ⓓ
7. Ⓐ Ⓑ Ⓒ Ⓓ	17. Ⓐ Ⓑ Ⓒ Ⓓ	27. Ⓐ Ⓑ Ⓒ Ⓓ
8. Ⓐ Ⓑ Ⓒ Ⓓ	18. Ⓐ Ⓑ Ⓒ Ⓓ	28. Ⓐ Ⓑ Ⓒ Ⓓ
9. Ⓐ Ⓑ Ⓒ Ⓓ	19. Ⓐ Ⓑ Ⓒ Ⓓ	29. Ⓐ Ⓑ Ⓒ Ⓓ
10. Ⓐ Ⓑ Ⓒ Ⓓ	20. Ⓐ Ⓑ Ⓒ Ⓓ	30. Ⓐ Ⓑ Ⓒ Ⓓ

Planning the Intervention

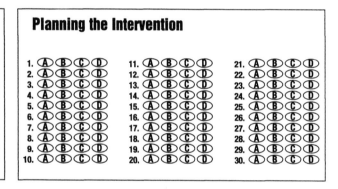

1. Ⓐ Ⓑ Ⓒ Ⓓ	11. Ⓐ Ⓑ Ⓒ Ⓓ	21. Ⓐ Ⓑ Ⓒ Ⓓ
2. Ⓐ Ⓑ Ⓒ Ⓓ	12. Ⓐ Ⓑ Ⓒ Ⓓ	22. Ⓐ Ⓑ Ⓒ Ⓓ
3. Ⓐ Ⓑ Ⓒ Ⓓ	13. Ⓐ Ⓑ Ⓒ Ⓓ	23. Ⓐ Ⓑ Ⓒ Ⓓ
4. Ⓐ Ⓑ Ⓒ Ⓓ	14. Ⓐ Ⓑ Ⓒ Ⓓ	24. Ⓐ Ⓑ Ⓒ Ⓓ
5. Ⓐ Ⓑ Ⓒ Ⓓ	15. Ⓐ Ⓑ Ⓒ Ⓓ	25. Ⓐ Ⓑ Ⓒ Ⓓ
6. Ⓐ Ⓑ Ⓒ Ⓓ	16. Ⓐ Ⓑ Ⓒ Ⓓ	26. Ⓐ Ⓑ Ⓒ Ⓓ
7. Ⓐ Ⓑ Ⓒ Ⓓ	17. Ⓐ Ⓑ Ⓒ Ⓓ	27. Ⓐ Ⓑ Ⓒ Ⓓ
8. Ⓐ Ⓑ Ⓒ Ⓓ	18. Ⓐ Ⓑ Ⓒ Ⓓ	28. Ⓐ Ⓑ Ⓒ Ⓓ
9. Ⓐ Ⓑ Ⓒ Ⓓ	19. Ⓐ Ⓑ Ⓒ Ⓓ	29. Ⓐ Ⓑ Ⓒ Ⓓ
10. Ⓐ Ⓑ Ⓒ Ⓓ	20. Ⓐ Ⓑ Ⓒ Ⓓ	30. Ⓐ Ⓑ Ⓒ Ⓓ

Implementing the Intervention

1. Ⓐ Ⓑ Ⓒ Ⓓ	11. Ⓐ Ⓑ Ⓒ Ⓓ	21. Ⓐ Ⓑ Ⓒ Ⓓ
2. Ⓐ Ⓑ Ⓒ Ⓓ	12. Ⓐ Ⓑ Ⓒ Ⓓ	22. Ⓐ Ⓑ Ⓒ Ⓓ
3. Ⓐ Ⓑ Ⓒ Ⓓ	13. Ⓐ Ⓑ Ⓒ Ⓓ	23. Ⓐ Ⓑ Ⓒ Ⓓ
4. Ⓐ Ⓑ Ⓒ Ⓓ	14. Ⓐ Ⓑ Ⓒ Ⓓ	24. Ⓐ Ⓑ Ⓒ Ⓓ
5. Ⓐ Ⓑ Ⓒ Ⓓ	15. Ⓐ Ⓑ Ⓒ Ⓓ	25. Ⓐ Ⓑ Ⓒ Ⓓ
6. Ⓐ Ⓑ Ⓒ Ⓓ	16. Ⓐ Ⓑ Ⓒ Ⓓ	26. Ⓐ Ⓑ Ⓒ Ⓓ
7. Ⓐ Ⓑ Ⓒ Ⓓ	17. Ⓐ Ⓑ Ⓒ Ⓓ	27. Ⓐ Ⓑ Ⓒ Ⓓ
8. Ⓐ Ⓑ Ⓒ Ⓓ	18. Ⓐ Ⓑ Ⓒ Ⓓ	28. Ⓐ Ⓑ Ⓒ Ⓓ
9. Ⓐ Ⓑ Ⓒ Ⓓ	19. Ⓐ Ⓑ Ⓒ Ⓓ	29. Ⓐ Ⓑ Ⓒ Ⓓ
10. Ⓐ Ⓑ Ⓒ Ⓓ	20. Ⓐ Ⓑ Ⓒ Ⓓ	30. Ⓐ Ⓑ Ⓒ Ⓓ

Documentation/Evaluation

1. Ⓐ Ⓑ Ⓒ Ⓓ	11. Ⓐ Ⓑ Ⓒ Ⓓ	21. Ⓐ Ⓑ Ⓒ Ⓓ
2. Ⓐ Ⓑ Ⓒ Ⓓ	12. Ⓐ Ⓑ Ⓒ Ⓓ	22. Ⓐ Ⓑ Ⓒ Ⓓ
3. Ⓐ Ⓑ Ⓒ Ⓓ	13. Ⓐ Ⓑ Ⓒ Ⓓ	23. Ⓐ Ⓑ Ⓒ Ⓓ
4. Ⓐ Ⓑ Ⓒ Ⓓ	14. Ⓐ Ⓑ Ⓒ Ⓓ	24. Ⓐ Ⓑ Ⓒ Ⓓ
5. Ⓐ Ⓑ Ⓒ Ⓓ	15. Ⓐ Ⓑ Ⓒ Ⓓ	25. Ⓐ Ⓑ Ⓒ Ⓓ
6. Ⓐ Ⓑ Ⓒ Ⓓ	16. Ⓐ Ⓑ Ⓒ Ⓓ	26. Ⓐ Ⓑ Ⓒ Ⓓ
7. Ⓐ Ⓑ Ⓒ Ⓓ	17. Ⓐ Ⓑ Ⓒ Ⓓ	27. Ⓐ Ⓑ Ⓒ Ⓓ
8. Ⓐ Ⓑ Ⓒ Ⓓ	18. Ⓐ Ⓑ Ⓒ Ⓓ	28. Ⓐ Ⓑ Ⓒ Ⓓ
9. Ⓐ Ⓑ Ⓒ Ⓓ	19. Ⓐ Ⓑ Ⓒ Ⓓ	29. Ⓐ Ⓑ Ⓒ Ⓓ
10. Ⓐ Ⓑ Ⓒ Ⓓ	20. Ⓐ Ⓑ Ⓒ Ⓓ	30. Ⓐ Ⓑ Ⓒ Ⓓ

Organizing/Managing

1. Ⓐ Ⓑ Ⓒ Ⓓ	11. Ⓐ Ⓑ Ⓒ Ⓓ	21. Ⓐ Ⓑ Ⓒ Ⓓ
2. Ⓐ Ⓑ Ⓒ Ⓓ	12. Ⓐ Ⓑ Ⓒ Ⓓ	22. Ⓐ Ⓑ Ⓒ Ⓓ
3. Ⓐ Ⓑ Ⓒ Ⓓ	13. Ⓐ Ⓑ Ⓒ Ⓓ	23. Ⓐ Ⓑ Ⓒ Ⓓ
4. Ⓐ Ⓑ Ⓒ Ⓓ	14. Ⓐ Ⓑ Ⓒ Ⓓ	24. Ⓐ Ⓑ Ⓒ Ⓓ
5. Ⓐ Ⓑ Ⓒ Ⓓ	15. Ⓐ Ⓑ Ⓒ Ⓓ	25. Ⓐ Ⓑ Ⓒ Ⓓ
6. Ⓐ Ⓑ Ⓒ Ⓓ	16. Ⓐ Ⓑ Ⓒ Ⓓ	26. Ⓐ Ⓑ Ⓒ Ⓓ
7. Ⓐ Ⓑ Ⓒ Ⓓ	17. Ⓐ Ⓑ Ⓒ Ⓓ	27. Ⓐ Ⓑ Ⓒ Ⓓ
8. Ⓐ Ⓑ Ⓒ Ⓓ	18. Ⓐ Ⓑ Ⓒ Ⓓ	28. Ⓐ Ⓑ Ⓒ Ⓓ
9. Ⓐ Ⓑ Ⓒ Ⓓ	19. Ⓐ Ⓑ Ⓒ Ⓓ	29. Ⓐ Ⓑ Ⓒ Ⓓ
10. Ⓐ Ⓑ Ⓒ Ⓓ	20. Ⓐ Ⓑ Ⓒ Ⓓ	30. Ⓐ Ⓑ Ⓒ Ⓓ

Advancement of the Profession

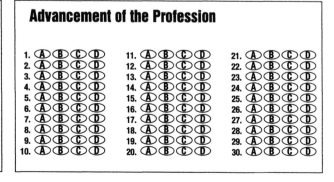

1. Ⓐ Ⓑ Ⓒ Ⓓ	11. Ⓐ Ⓑ Ⓒ Ⓓ	21. Ⓐ Ⓑ Ⓒ Ⓓ
2. Ⓐ Ⓑ Ⓒ Ⓓ	12. Ⓐ Ⓑ Ⓒ Ⓓ	22. Ⓐ Ⓑ Ⓒ Ⓓ
3. Ⓐ Ⓑ Ⓒ Ⓓ	13. Ⓐ Ⓑ Ⓒ Ⓓ	23. Ⓐ Ⓑ Ⓒ Ⓓ
4. Ⓐ Ⓑ Ⓒ Ⓓ	14. Ⓐ Ⓑ Ⓒ Ⓓ	24. Ⓐ Ⓑ Ⓒ Ⓓ
5. Ⓐ Ⓑ Ⓒ Ⓓ	15. Ⓐ Ⓑ Ⓒ Ⓓ	25. Ⓐ Ⓑ Ⓒ Ⓓ
6. Ⓐ Ⓑ Ⓒ Ⓓ	16. Ⓐ Ⓑ Ⓒ Ⓓ	26. Ⓐ Ⓑ Ⓒ Ⓓ
7. Ⓐ Ⓑ Ⓒ Ⓓ	17. Ⓐ Ⓑ Ⓒ Ⓓ	27. Ⓐ Ⓑ Ⓒ Ⓓ
8. Ⓐ Ⓑ Ⓒ Ⓓ	18. Ⓐ Ⓑ Ⓒ Ⓓ	28. Ⓐ Ⓑ Ⓒ Ⓓ
9. Ⓐ Ⓑ Ⓒ Ⓓ	19. Ⓐ Ⓑ Ⓒ Ⓓ	29. Ⓐ Ⓑ Ⓒ Ⓓ
10. Ⓐ Ⓑ Ⓒ Ⓓ	20. Ⓐ Ⓑ Ⓒ Ⓓ	30. Ⓐ Ⓑ Ⓒ Ⓓ

Diagnostic and Review Items
Answer Scoring Key

Background

1. A	11. A	21. C
2. B	12. C	22. D
3. C	13. C	23. D
4. A	14. C	24. C
5. A	15. D	25. A
6. C	16. A	26. D
7. C	17. B	27. C
8. A	18. A	28. A
9. B	19. A	29. B
10. A	20. B	30. A

Diagnostic Groupings

1. C	11. B	21. C
2. A	12. A	22. A
3. A	13. B	23. B
4. B	14. D	24. C
5. B	15. A	25. D
6. A	16. C	26. D
7. B	17. D	27. D
8. C	18. B	28. B
9. C	19. C	29. B
10. B	20. A	30. B

Assessment

1. B	11. B	21. A
2. B	12. D	22. B
3. D	13. A	23. A
4. A	14. D	24. A
5. D	15. A	25. D
6. B	16. D	26. C
7. D	17. B	27. A
8. B	18. D	28. D
9. A	19. B	29. A
10. B	20. A	30. A

Planning the Intervention

1. B	11. A	21. D
2. A	12. D	22. D
3. C	13. B	23. B
4. D	14. A	24. A
5. A	15. A	25. C
6. A	16. A	26. D
7. B	17. B	27. B
8. D	18. C	28. C
9. D	19. B	29. C
10. B	20. B	30. C

Implementing the Intervention

1. **D**	11. **D**	21. **C**
2. **A**	12. **A**	22. **A**
3. **D**	13. **A**	23. **C**
4. **B**	14. **D**	24. **B**
5. **A**	15. **A**	25. **A**
6. **C**	16. **A**	26. **A**
7. **C**	17. **C**	27. **B**
8. **B**	18. **A**	28. **B**
9. **A**	19. **D**	29. **C**
10. **B**	20. **A**	30. **D**

Documentation/Evaluation

1. **D**	11. **A**	21. **A**
2. **A**	12. **A**	22. **A**
3. **D**	13. **A**	23. **A**
4. **D**	14. **A**	24. **C**
5. **C**	15. **B**	25. **A**
6. **B**	16. **D**	26. **A**
7. **B**	17. **B**	27. **D**
8. **A**	18. **C**	28. **A**
9. **B**	19. **D**	29. **C**
10. **C**	20. **B**	30. **C**

Organizing/Managing

1. **A**	11. **A**	21. **A**
2. **A**	12. **D**	22. **C**
3. **A**	13. **A**	23. **C**
4. **C**	14. **A**	24. **B**
5. **B**	15. **C**	25. **D**
6. **C**	16. **C**	26. **B**
7. **C**	17. **B**	27. **C**
8. **A**	18. **A**	28. **D**
9. **D**	19. **C**	29. **B**
10. **D**	20. **C**	30. **D**

Advancement of the Profession

1. **B**	11. **B**	21. **D**
2. **D**	12. **A**	22. **B**
3. **A**	13. **A**	23. **C**
4. **C**	14. **D**	24. **C**
5. **A**	15. **B**	25. **C**
6. **C**	16. **C**	26. **D**
7. **A**	17. **D**	27. **C**
8. **A**	18. **B**	28. **B**
9. **C**	19. **C**	29. **C**
10. **B**	20. **C**	30. **A**